41.66

OPEN WIDER
Your Wallet, Not Your Mouth

Everything you need to
know when you visit the dentist

A Consumer's Guide To Dentistry

Fred Quarnstrom, DDS

D1157319

APR 14 2009

Dedication

To my patients from whom I have learned.

To all the dentists who have treated us and others fairly, with skill and dedication.

To our spouses, our best friends, who have put up with our many evenings at the computer producing this book.

Table of Contents

I. Are you in good hands?

HERMAN®

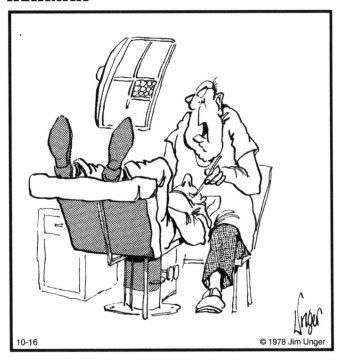

10-16 © 1978 Jim Unger

**"Dentistry's come a long way
in the last few years."**

1. Become a smart dental consumer

*"Of course you need an
aesthetic makeover.
You need 20 crowns.
You will be more beautiful.
You will have more friends.
You will be more successful;
And, I need a new car."*

The dentist/barber

It used to be you went to a dentist/barber when you had a toothache. He (because it was mostly men back then) fixed whatever was wrong or removed the offending tooth, and that was that. There was no glamour to it, just a utilitarian profession that focused on relieving pain. Barbers gave way to dentists. In the early days one dentist taught another to be a dentist. It was an apprentice system. This gave way to formal dental schools. In time, the emphasis went to saving teeth. By doing fillings, pain and infections were avoided, and people chewed better.

Dentures were the norm

However, everyone knew they would eventually wear dentures. Even 40 years ago at least 50% of the population wore dentures by the time they retired.

How you looked after dental treatment was a secondary consideration. We only had gold and silver fillings. It was common to see patients with gold in the front of the mouth. The dentists weren't particularly rich and weren't expected to be. They did what their patients needed and in doing so they could expect a good, if not an opulent, life.

Marketing is now the emphasis of some dentists

How the field of dentistry has changed! Once a dentist graduates, a lot of time is spent learning how to maximize profits. Marketing appeals to the cosmetic aspects of dentistry rather than medical needs. Dentistry is becoming a lot like hairdressing or artificial nails, with patients making choices for aesthetics rather than medical reasons. That's not bad in itself. In fact, looking good has definite benefits, and if that's what you want, then by all means, go for it. But do so for the right reasons, and make sure the right person works on your mouth. In this book we will help you choose the right dentist, and the treatment that is right for you.

A good dentist can make you smile with confidence. But the problem is, it is now so easy to be oversold. Some treatments that are pushed as necessary in fact aren't. Others promise to do a lot more for you than they can deliver.

Rich folks are taken advantage of

Did you know that people in affluent

neighborhoods have substantially more dental procedures than people in less wealthy areas? Where you live is the most valid predictor of what your dental needs will be, or more accurately, what will be sold to you as opposed to your actual needs.

Isn't it surprising, considering how much more resources the affluent people have to take better care of themselves? But when you look deeper, it is not surprising at all. Why set up in a poor community if there are wealthy communities? Many dentists to the wealthy have advertising budgets of $300,000 per year or more. And someone has to pay for it one way or another. Don't let that be you.

We need to become careful consumers. Because of my unpleasant experiences in the past, I now ask questions and am rigorous in trusting my instincts as I enter a new relationship with anyone in dentistry, and in any medical field for that matter. I have learned through observation. I have learned from my mistakes.

Some of the best most cost-effective dentistry comes out of small towns and older, modest income neighborhoods. The people in these areas are prudent consumers. They question the need for everything that is done because the cost is significant to them and their families. They essentially train the dentists. They do not let the dentist overtreat because they will ask about it. The other issue is that those inclined to overtreat or specialize in "aesthetic dentistry" quickly leave these areas because these patients will not tolerate this form of dentistry.

Anne's story

I grew up with the same dentist. He was conservative and careful. He regarded his patients as his family and he took good care of all of us. There were many times that I left his exam room needing no work. He had emergency coverage when he was out of town. I assumed all dentists had this protection for their patients. That is not the case. It pays to ask questions and investigate office policies before you need help and can't find it.

I then moved to California. I went to a dentist's office and after my first appointment they sent me flowers and the person who referred me a dozen roses. Does that pass the common sense test? I don't think so. And guess who ultimately pays for all that stuff? Wouldn't you rather they used that money on training and equipment?

I have watched the proliferation of cosmetic dentistry and marketing and I have wondered how the consumer can find the level of care they are personally comfortable with. Times are changing. So, we have tried to put together a guide to the profession that will allow you to advocate for your own dental health.

My red flag system

When I seek a new caregiver I ask for their qualifications. I do this before I make an appointment. I look around to see what they are selling in the waiting room. If I get far enough to go in for a cleaning appointment, I ask the hygienist if they are paid based upon the services they sell while they are working on my mouth. Plus, when I have a new dentist who recommends aggressive treatment, I get a second opinion. If seeking another opinion bothers them, that is a huge red flag.

Hopefully, this book will help you to develop your own red flag system. We have made an attempt to help you have more information about how to take care of your dental health.

The second patient's bad experience (Marzena's story)

I have two reasons for wanting to be involved with this book. First is my own experience, so let me share it. Second is my friend's experience, which I will also share.

I can't claim a dazzling smile, but I have always tried to take good care of my teeth. Many of them have fillings, but they serve me well. I brush regularly, although I confess I don't floss every day.

It was right after I moved to the Seattle area. I had a brand new dental insurance and decided to use it by getting my teeth cleaned. Since I was new to the area, I didn't really know anyone to ask for a recommendation. I picked a dentist that was close to where I worked and made an appointment.

The spa practice

The office was elegant and well appointed. The dentist was pleasant in an impersonal kind of way, but I figured I didn't need him to be my best friend, so that was fine with me. He carefully examined my teeth, and nodded sadly. Then to my complete shock he announced that my mouth was a complete mess! I needed extensive dental work, including numerous new crowns. My fillings were all failing, requiring immediate replacement.

I listened in horror. Visions of a toothless smile appeared in my head. The dentist suggested helpfully that he would create a treatment plan for me so we could get the work done in a methodical way, starting immediately. I tried asking some questions but didn't get good answers. The gist of it was that he was an expert, and he expected me to follow his recommendation because I didn't know much about teeth.

I left, puzzled and worried. But after the original shock had passed, I started thinking clearly. I was getting more than a little annoyed. How could it be? Not so long ago I had gone to my regular dentist, and my teeth were just fine. Yes, I had a lot of fillings, and some of them were old. I knew they might fail at some point, but why would they all fail at the same time? I might not be an expert on dentistry, but I'm no dummy. I have a good brain and I know how to use it. The dentist should have made some effort to explain his recommendations. I decided I wasn't having anything done that I didn't fully understand. I would find another dentist.

But I had a new job, and soon I was too busy to think about such trivia as my teeth. As is often the case, fate intervened. I woke up one Saturday with a toothache. To make matters worse, it was a long weekend, and many dental offices were closed.

Yet another dentist

I remembered my less than successful visit at the first dentist and I had no intention of going back. I still didn't know many people here other than my coworkers, who by now were enjoying their long weekend. So, I had nobody to ask for recommendations, again. But this time I resolved I was going to get smarter. I would not rely on the good old phone book. I remembered the ads for 1-800-DENTIST. The ads promised to put me in touch with a qualified dentist, not just with anybody. The dentists were screened and approved. How could I lose?

I picked up the phone and dialed the number. A nice lady at the other end listened sympathetically, asked me a few questions, and made an appointment for me.

You pay more downtown

The office was in a beautiful building right downtown. It offered valet parking, and other amenities I wouldn't normally expect of a dentist. I was a little worried that they would be very expensive, but after all I had a good dental insurance. Surely, it would cover my emergency.

The first thing the nice receptionist wanted from me was my credit card. I explained that I had insurance and it covered a lot of the costs. Still, they would charge my credit card with some of the costs, and they would credit it back later. Exhausted from pain, I agreed.

The scam

I don't remember exactly what they did, but the pain did go away. I went home happy and was even happier that my insurance covered the whole thing. But to my annoyance I found that my credit card had been charged $50. That wasn't a huge amount as dental fees go, but mine was supposed to be all covered! Plus, it was my money and I was entitled to have it. I phoned the dentist and was told that they would keep the money toward the cost of my next visit. It didn't matter what I said, they just wouldn't refund it.

So, I had two experiences with American dentists, both of them bad. It was time to get serious and find myself a dentist I could trust.

About that time, my husband and I bought our first house. Seattle is expensive, and we couldn't afford a beautiful house in an affluent neighborhood, but we did find a nice small house in a pleasant part of town. We asked our new neighbors about a good dentist, and the same name kept coming up. I went on the Web and found out that Dr Q had ties to the University of Washington. I made the appointment.

The office of Dr Q was clean and practical. There were no posh decorations here. The staff was multiracial, reflecting the ethnic character of the neighborhood. Dr Q took time to carefully answer all my questions until I fully understood. No, my mouth was not a mess. My old fillings were fine, and I was doing a good job at keeping my teeth clean. Yes, some teeth possibly could use crowns, but it was not absolutely necessary and certainly not urgent. I was deathly afraid of crowns, partly because of the pain I imagined it would cause, and partly because the process is irreversible. Dr Q patiently explained that many dentists considered it a standard practice to crown all teeth that had root canals. That was not a practice where I had come from, and we agreed not to do anything drastic right then. I felt relieved and comfortable with my new dentist. (I have let Dr Q put a crown on one of my teeth since.)

I also shared the story of overcharging and was told such a practice was illegal. He suggested I phone that dentist and threaten to report them if my money was not refunded. I did so and got the money back immediately. Funny how a little knowledge of your rights can make such a huge difference.

A friend's experience

I mentioned two reasons for being involved in this book. One is the experience I described above. The other is my friend. She is a charming, attractive woman, but for some reason she didn't like the way she looked. Her husband had some business ties to a cosmetic dentist who offered to correct her smile for a large discount. Her jaw was supposedly constructed in such a way that she risked severe headaches later.

We suggested that it was not that obvious the headaches would come, and if they did, they could be treated then. She was attractive, and we didn't see why she should go ahead with such a radical treatment. But she decided to go for it, partly out of concern for the headaches, partly out of a desire for a nicer smile.

It took months and months of braces, followed by a jaw surgery, followed by yet more months of braces. Two years and many thousands of dollars later she didn't look much different.

I hope this book helps someone facing difficult decisions like that. I am not against cosmetic dentistry. But I am against dishonest dentists who try to reach deeply into pockets of unsuspected patients, abusing their position of power and getting rich at the expense of people who don't have the knowledge to protect themselves. This book will offer you the knowledge to protect yourself and your loved ones.

When I hear stories like this I always remember a tee shirt I once saw. It said, "Trust me, I am a doctor." There was a time when this was prudent. No longer. If a dentist tells you your fillings are all failing and you have had no problems in the past few years, be cautious. One of the biggest indicators to replace fillings is going to a new dentist. If you visited your old dentist regularly, and all was well, there is no need to change. If the new dentist suggests that you need to remove all the alloys (silver fillings) and replace them with tooth-colored fillings, be especially cautious. If they tell you the silver fillings are 50% mercury (which is true) and then tell you mercury is a poison (which is true but the mercury is bound in the silver and can not be released without heating the fillings to about 400 degrees) run, do not walk, to the door. No one has ever been harmed by silver fillings. If you want tooth-colored fillings, that is your choice. But realize that we know they will not last as well as silver. Tooth-colored fillings will look much nicer. You can be beautiful for 10 years or ugly for the rest of your life (with silver fillings) hopefully only in back.

An old beat up chipped filling may be the best. If they got that old, they were well done and if left alone can well last for many more years. If they fail, break, or get decay, you can have them replaced then.

Dental referral services charge dentists large fees, often per each patient referred. This has not worked well for dentists because most of the patients referred are emergencies that only want a tooth pulled and have little interest in doing fillings or other work to prevent emergencies in the future. The cost of the service often is equal to the fees for an extraction.

Jaw surgery is major surgery. There is a real risk of death from general anesthesia. It is possible that you can end up with a numb lower jaw. The absolutely worst outcome can be death of major areas of bone. I have heard of cases where a large part of the upper jaw was lost along with 6 or 8 front teeth.

If you are not having headaches, it is very doubtful if anyone can predict they will happen if you do not choose to undergo the jaw surgery. There is a real risk that if you disrupt the relationship between upper and lower jaws that you can have such problems.

2. Who looks out for the patient?

The physics professor is your friend

There is an old joke about a pre-dental student in a college physics class. He protested that physics was something he would never use again, was a waste of time, and would not make him a better dentist. The professor said, "Do not be so sure. This class saves lives."

Puzzled, the student responded, "How could this class save lives?"

The professor responded, "It keeps idiots like you out of medical and dental school."

Admission to dental school

In fact, the physics professor might have more to do with the competence of your dentist than anyone. It has become increasingly difficult to get into dental school. Several deans brag that they could not get into their own dental school if they were to apply today with their pre-dental school grades. It is not unusual for the entering freshman class of a dental school to have an average GPA in excess of 3.7 out of a possible 4.0. Thirty years ago you could get in with a 3.0, or even a little lower. There has been some grade inflation since, so it is not fair to compare the two figures directly, but still, today's figure is impressive. Most, if not all, of each class will have a degree and 4 years of undergraduate school. Many will have 5 years of college.

The admission process is a bit more complex too. There is an interview now that was not done when I was admitted. I am not convinced this is of much value. One student I know who applied was only asked two or three questions and then dismissed. He clearly had not impressed the interviewer. I heard of the problem and found a person to help him practice for a new interview. I heard later that the turning point in his second interview came when he described keeping one of his friends awake and walking one night after the friend took a drug overdose. This somehow indicated he was more in touch with society and would be a better dentist. It must be true, as he was accepted, graduated, and has been in practice for over 15 years and is providing good care for his patients.

Dental school

Once you get in, the next hurdle in becoming a dentist is the 4 years of dental school. Thirty years ago they would accept 75 students knowing that they would probably not graduate more than 55. That system was not fair. There were many good dentists who did not graduate because it took them a little longer to master some skill. If you failed one class, you were out. You could not retake the class. If you got 2 Ds, you were out

Everyone assumes that some time is spent teaching ethics to dental school and that is true, kind of—they have a short class the second quarter of their senior year. Of course, ethics should be a topic from day one. In fact, some of the students complain that some of the requirements they must complete to graduate compromise their ethics.

Procedure requirements

Here is what they mean. Each student must do a specific number of procedures in each area of dentistry to graduate. For example, they will need to do 5 gold crowns or inlays. Many teeth have perfectly good silver fillings removed and replaced with the crown or inlay so a student can meet their graduation requirement. Many of these teeth would go years and would require no treatment.

The ethics class then tries to convince students it is unethical to overtreat, just when they have been told by instructors that they should replace adequate silver fillings with gold crowns and inlays.

It is rare today to have any student flunk or be forced out of school. A few will decide on their own that it is not for them, or they are not up to the pressure they must endure. The classes are brutal. A normal college load for a quarter would be 15 credit hours of courses for a quarter. This would be 3 hours of lecture a day 5 days a week. In contrast, dental schools often have 20 to 22 credit hours per quarter. One quarter we had 27 credit hours. We were in school from 8

AM to 4PM or later every day. We went home to hours of reading or lab work to prepare for the next day. So dental school is a hurdle you must complete. If you are admitted, you will probably graduate. You are reasonably smart or you would not have been accepted to dental school.

Licensing boards

Next, you must take a board exam. Written national board exams occur at the end of the second year of dental school and in the senior year. They cover the academic portions of dental school. It sounds like a good program. However, when I took the test, each student was assigned a question to memorize while taking the test. These questions were collected by the class and sold as a study guide to the next year's class. So each student can easily have two or three old tests to serve as a study guide. Unethical, yes, but that's a typical practice. For this reason, it is unusual for a student to fail national boards.

The practical portion of the dental boards is a test on actual patients. It is administered by each state. Many states band together to give regional boards. There are three or four such major boards and an attempt is being made to make a national test. Some states accept only their own boards; other states will accept the boards of most other states. In general, to take the boards you must be a graduate of an American or Canadian dental school. All foreign graduates must complete at least 2 years in an American or Canadian dental school. There is talk of certifying some of the Mexican dental schools. The Governor of each state appoints the licensing/disciplinary Board members. They usually are picked from a pool nominated by the state dental society.

Board candidates are expected to bring 3 or 4 patients to the board exam. They will perform a specific dental procedure on those patients. Often this includes doing a silver filling, a gold inlay, cleaning part of the mouth, doing a root canal on an extracted tooth, and other procedures depending on the board.

Some students fail because of the patients they selected. If the patient does not show on the appointed day, you fail. If the patient is fidgety at the wrong time or cannot tolerate being in the exam situation, you fail. Ditto if there is an undetectable defect in the tooth that prevents you from doing the test procedure. Say you wanted to do a silver filling, but the decay is more extensive than it appeared and you must do a crown. You fail, because you were asked to show your competency at doing a silver filling.

One thing that has improved is that board examiners now get together and practice. Their grading is better calibrated and is much better documented.

Is the fact that the prospective dentist passed the board a guarantee to the patient? Probably not as much as the fact that they graduated from an accredited school. Is this to say that foreign schools are all bad? No. However, many of the third world countries' dental schools are really substandard. Patients really do need to be protected from these graduates. On the other hand, there are many foreign schools that do turn out well-qualified dentists who have a very difficult time becoming certified to practice in the US.

The physics professor may be the key

So what part of this system does the most to ensure a well-trained dentist? That physics professor may, in fact, be the best predictor of their competence. Pre-dental school grades need to be almost perfect. A "B" in a physics or chemistry class may be the biggest hurtle to substandard students.

A license is forever

Once a dentist passes the boards and has a license, provided they do not do something very bad, like forcing sex on a patient, they are set for life. It is nearly impossible to lose a dental license. A license is considered personal property. In cases of impropriety, fraud, and the like, a dentist might lose the license for 5 years and then the board will place a requirement on the dentist to get it back. The dentist might have to go through continuing education, rehabilitation or counseling, and might have to retake the boards.

The states do talk to each other, but this takes time. If a dentist has a license restricted in one state, they can simply move to another state. In time, often a year or so, the new state will find out the dentist lost the license in the first state and they will often restrict the license also. The restricting state may not know there is a license in another state. The second state will find out but it will take time.

What mechanisms are in place to protect the patient from a dentist who either sneaks past the admission committee, dental school professors, and the boards? Fortunately most dentists are honest, hard working folks who truly do their best. But it still makes sense for you to guard against some bad apples that unfortunately are out there.

How to protect yourself

Prevention may be your best guide. Go to the website of your particular state licensing board and check out your dentist. This is very easy in some states. California has a very user friendly site. The state of Washington has a site that is very difficult to use and you get very little information unless there has been a major problem. Has your dentist come before the board? What were the circumstances? If you have insurance and your dentist's treatment keeps being rejected, be on guard. It may be you are requesting treatment for aesthetic reasons that are usually not covered. It may be that the dentist is requesting treatment that is not indicated.

What if you have a complaint?

Peer review

Patients who feel, for whatever reason, they were mistreated have several avenues open to them. The first and easiest is to go to the local dental association. Most have a peer review committee. While this committee is made up of practicing dentists and can only review those dentists who are members of the dental society, this mechanism does not cost anything and often can resolve problems. Most problems have to do with fees.

I served on our local peer review committee for several years. Often you could come to a compromise because it was easier for the dentist to give in than take a chance on a malpractice suit or a trip to the licensing commission or board. It simply was less costly to agree to a patient's demands than it was to take the time to answer them.

The disciplinary board

For cases that are more serious, dentists that are not members of the dental society and where a compromise cannot be reached, there is the Dental Disciplinary Board or Quality Assurance

Commission. These are state appointed boards. Most are composed of dentists and usually include laypersons. The dentists are usually nominated by the dental association but are appointed by the Governor in most states. Some states are clearly "good old boy/girl clubs." The joke is if you are not having sex with the Governor's spouse you will not be disciplined.

The boards/commissions have the ultimate solution to problems—they can revoke a dentist's license. Without a license a dental degree is of little value. The boards and commissions, as you see, are not perfect. The process clearly protects the dentist in that the dentist is presumed innocent and it is the state that must prove they are guilty. If a commission member is familiar with a case, they will probably be removed from that case because of their knowledge. If a case appears to be difficult, it might be dropped or an attempt to settle it will be a high priority. Difficult cases take time, money, and resources. The boards and/or commissions will be pressured to settle cases quickly and easily. The state personnel are under less pressure to prosecute than they are under pressure to have a balanced budget.

The process is not the same in each state. First, call the state's dental licensing board. Many states will follow something like the following mechanism. Ask for a complaint form. You will next be asked if they can release your name.

Most states have whistle blower statutes that allow you to not release your name. However, if you do not release your name, they cannot ask for a copy of your records and the complaint ends.

If you will not release your name, the investigations cannot go ahead. The investigators cannot go to an office and examine random charts. Even dentists are considered to be innocent until proven guilty. Without a complaint they cannot be investigated.

If you do allow your name to be used, your complaint will go to a committee, usually consisting of board members who will not be allowed to know your name or the dentist's name. They will look at your complaint and decide whether it should be investigated. Some complaints will not be investigated. Here is the list of these that will differ from state to state:

- Fee disputes. Some of these will be investigated, but often there is a minimum below which they will not investigate.
- Suits to recover money.
- Those dentists that are not licensed.
- Insurance issues.
- Rudeness of the dentist or their staff.
- Miscommunication.

If you have any of the above problems, you should file the complaint anyway; all it costs is a stamp. There might be other problems with this dentist that you do not know about and that might trigger an investigation.

Many boards will not look at issues that are below a certain amount of money. But they are becoming very alert and sensitive to substance abuse, sexual impropriety, dirty offices, and procedural lapses such as lack of gloves and masks.

Once a complaint is heard by this committee it will either be dropped (rare for our commission) or sent on for investigation. The state has a number of investigators. Investigation can be as simple as asking for a copy of all your records, including your x-rays.

What if your dentist alters your records? This is a very silly thing to do and it is usually pretty easy to detect. Altering records is a serious offense that can lead to loss of license. It is therefore extremely unlikely that you will face this type of offense. Most dental records are not very complete and many are close to impossible to read unless you are clairvoyant.

If the complaint is sent for investigation, records are collected, the patient will be interviewed, and the dentist might be interviewed (by this time they should have called their insurance company and an attorney usually steps in and prevents this interview.) The file is turned over to one of the commission members who will review all the records. It is not unusual to have several hundreds of pages. That reviewing commission member will go before a panel of the board with a summary of the case and a recommendation as to what should be done.

In one case, a patient came to me for sedation. He had been our patient for about 5 years. He moved 50 miles away and found a local dentist who would use oral sedation. We had never needed more that 0.5mg, two tablets, of halcion to treat him. He was always awake and cooperative.

The new dentist gave him 10 tablets. Fortunately his sister-in-law was a registered nurse. She stayed with him for 24 hours making sure he was breathing. He would stop breathing if she stopped talking to him or pinching him. It was a very dangerous situation and tragedy was avoided only because of her nursing background. She made him come back to us for his next treatment.

I videotaped the session in which I used 2 tablets. He was a large person around 240 lbs. I filed a complaint with our Dental Quality Assurance Commission. I sent the video and copies of his records along with a narrative that explained why what the previous dentist had done was so dangerous. The only way the documentation could have been better would have been if the commission had actually been in the room and if they had followed the patient home.

Because I had filed the complaint with the commission, I could not sit in on the discussion. I knew too much, how close the patient had been to a disaster, and just how dangerous the other dentist's dose had been. People have committed suicide with such a dose. This was a very lucky patient to have survived his appointment.

The reviewing commission member presented the case to the panel, and because of his synopsis of the case, they all decided this treatment was within standard of care. This process protects the dentist but does nothing to protect his patients.

If you have a commission member who knows a topic, does research in the topic, publishes on oral conscious sedation, it makes no sense to not take any advice from the expert. However, the protection of this dangerous dentist was placed above that of his patient.

There can be one of several outcomes. The case can be dropped. It can be referred back for more investigation. The case can go to a settlement conference to be referred for mediation to determine if a settlement can be reached. Or it can be referred for a statement of charges.

In the case of a settlement, the commission member, the dentist, an attorney for state, and an attorney for the dentist will meet. A settlement will be attempted. Often this includes a fine and requirement for additional training for the dentist, and possibly the state will demand practice restrictions. Of course, the dentist and his attorney will attempt to negotiate a lower level of penalty. If no compromise is possible, the case will usually go to a statement of charges.

In a recent case of some very bad treatment by a dentist, I negotiated a $40,000 fine. The dentist had to return all fees to the Patients and their insurance company. The dentist was required to *attend 60 hours of hands-on training. I intended for the dentist to employ a specialist to examine his work, teach him, and review the dentistry being preformed and then for the specialist to give us a report on the dentist's level of competence. The attorneys got involved and because of the way the state's attorneys wrote up the case, the dentist was able to just attend a course where he did some work on plastic models.*

There is a risk that the dentist will go to a continuing education (CE) course, sit in the back of the room, and learn nothing. The legal documents did not state the course had to be hands-on. They did state that I had to approve of the courses; I had to approve the course and refused to do so. It was not the course we had agreed to in the settlement conference. I was told by the state to either approve the course or the state would give it to a different commission member and they would approve it. I did not feel it fair to dump this on someone else, so I gave in to the state. The state was clearly more worried about the dentist than they were about the patient.

It should be mentioned that this dentist was restricted from doing anything but the simplest procedures until he had completed all his courses and paid his fine. He was not allowed to do any of the procedures he had problems doing until he had taken the required CE courses.

It was less costly for the State to just accept the CE. It really did not matter that the courses were the same courses he had taken before. I will know better next time. All future settlements will be very specific of the type of course needed.

The joke (it is not funny) is that some of the bad dentists have had so much CE they are about to qualify for an advanced degree in that aspect of dentistry. They have been back to the board 5, 10, or even 15 times. The continuing education has had no effect. I found dental school professors who were willing to do hands-on training and evaluation. However, the State and the dental school have taken two years and have yet to agree to this program. The individual professors are willing, only the lack of cooperation between the school and the state is holding this up. In the mean time, the continuing education requirements are a laugh. The continuing education courses have not been successful in the past to change the actions of the wayward dentists. Does it sound like the commission is really looking out for the patients or is it more interested in the dentist having an easy time out of meaningless classes?

If the settlement conference is not successful or if the violation is very serious the next step is for the state attorneys to file a statement of charges (SOC). Both sides gather expert witnesses and the case is heard in front of a panel of the board with a judge, court reporters and attorneys for both sides. These cases can run several days to several weeks. They are quite costly for the state and the dentist, or at least the dentist's insurance company. The patient will usually be one of the witnesses. The finding of the court will be released in 120 days. This is really unfortunate because the decision is made at the end of the hearing. The dentist continues to practice until several months later when the outcome is made public. If a license is to be pulled it should be pulled immediately.

I have an impression from working on our commission that in some cases the state intercedes in this process and attempts to interfere to save money when a case will be difficult to prove. Certainly in several of my cases, state middle management attempted to browbeat me into accepting compromises that let the dentist off with a hand slap. In one case of a death, they refused to reopen a case when new information came to light. The state feared a drawn out legal challenge by the dentist's attorney.

There was more concern about the budget than protecting patients. Middle management used several tactics; they were too busy to look at all these cases, recommended to just give more continuing education, and didn't think it mattered that the dentist had taken this course before with no effect; the state may be sued if they try to reopen the death case. Heavy-handed attempts were taken to make me accept sanctions that were less than a slap on the hand.

If your dentist has multiple violations, be a little careful, but it doesn't necessarily mean the dentist did something wrong. Find out what the violations were. For example, some patients will develop an allergy to penicillin midway through a course of antibiotics, and there is no way to prevent this. Some states require that a dentist turn themselves in to the board/ commission if they send a patient to a hospital. In my 42 year long career, I have sent 4 patients to a hospital: 2 for allergies, and two because they came to the office with severe infections that required hospitalization. All 4 were treated appropriately and it was good dentistry to send them to the hospital, but they show as closed violations because I sent patients to a hospital. This is a stupid regulation. We should modify it. If the patient ends up in the hospital because of something the dentist did wrong, that is a different matter.

While I believe all persons, even dentists, are innocent until proven guilty, I think the patient's rights and protection come first. The legal system is a major deterrent to the disciplinary system. Because the license is considered personal property, it is very difficult to remove. If you are about to lose your license, your way to make a living is threatened, so you will hire the most high-powered attorney money can buy. The same is true for expert witnesses. The state's attorneys have large case loads and are simply outgunned many times. As a friend who is an attorney stated, "I love to go against an attorney who works 9 to 5."

We had one dentist who had been before the board 17 times. Each trip was a new event and the board was not allowed to know about the other cases. Many were money issues that were below threshold. If you rip off a patient for $3000 you might be sanctioned, but if you rip off 10 patients for $800 each you will not be because none of the amounts reached that unpublished threshold. This is a bit like saying if you kill someone with a single bullet to the heart you will be judged, but if you use a shot gun you can get off because none of the individual pellets would be lethal. This particular dentist figured out how to work the system by the legal constraints of not letting the board know of previous cases.

What if a dentist prescribes thousands of dollars of unnecessary dentistry? I have seen cases where a patient goes to a dentist who produces a treatment plan for $30,000 or $40,000 of crowns and veneers. The patient is suspicious and sees a second dentist who says none of it is necessary. Do you think the first dentist will be sanctioned? No, because nothing happened to the patient. The work was never done.

I was shocked the first time such a case came before the board I was sitting on, and the answer was that the first dentist did not do any work, so he could not be charged with overtreatment. I think this is very short-sighted. The only reason the overtreatment didn't happen was that the patient was wise enough to get a second opinion. I feel that presenting a case and suggesting that unnecessary work should be done is almost as bad as doing unnecessary work.

Sexual misadventures

How effective are state regulatory boards?

Let's take a look as several cases I am familiar with. A dentist was arrested and charged in court with molesting a female patient while she was under the effect of nitrous oxide sedation. She claimed she woke up in a staff lounge undressed with the dentist pulling up his pants. There was some question if the sedative gas was potent enough for this to happen. The dentist claimed they had just had consensual union. The fact that they were both married to other folks did not seem to bother him. The case became the focus of the local newspaper. As I remember he was not convicted in court but certainly was in the press. His license remained in effect. Having sex, consensual or otherwise, does not necessarily result in revocation of one's license.

How about pedophilia? A dentist was accused before the licensing board and confessed to making advances to young boys while in his office. He was found guilty by the board and they lifted his right to treat children without having a third person in the treatment room. As it turns out, pedophilia was not considered reason to revoke a license.

Breast massage

A more recent case was a dentist treating women who had tempormandibular, facial, pain. He started massaging their facial muscles that were in spasm. He proceeded to massage the woman's neck muscles that might have also been in spasm. Up to this point the therapy might have been appropriate. However, when he went on to massage the patient's breasts, it became very difficult to show a dental connection. His license was rescinded for a number of years. He went off to practice in another state. That license was rescinded in the new state and he came back and appealed our original decision to a superior court. The court sent the case back to the commission for a new hearing. The outcome of the second hearing was the same. It will now go back to the superior court judge. He has appealed this case one more time. The good news is, he is not practicing while all this takes place. However, the new judge could give him his license back. His next move was to threaten the state and every member of the commission with multimillion dollar law suits if we did not drop the sanction. As Yogi Bera said, "It ain't over till it's over."

Alcohol abuse

One dentist who lost his license did so after arriving in the office under the influence of alcohol five times. Once should be enough, certainly two or three times is adequate. Another interesting case has to do with a dentist who wrote prescriptions for his staff and family, first for antibiotics to treat acne. Later he went on to prescribe medication for various minor gynecological problems and finally narcotic pain medication for himself. He received a slap on the hand and a fine. He was not stopped from advertising for new business. All you had to do was pick up the Sunday newspaper supplement or several other magazines to find his ad proposing he was an expert in giving you a perfect smile. He even was cited by *Seattle Magazine* as being one of the area's most outstanding dentists. Did his full-page ad in that magazine have anything to do with the selection? Did the magazine bother to check him out with the state board?

Fraud

Fraud should get bad dentists stripped of their licenses. I reviewed a case where a dentist charged for five 3/4 gold crowns at a cost of about $4000. I had the patient go to a respected senior dentist who taught part time in a dental school. He called me most upset. There were no gold crowns or even gold inlays in the patient's mouth. There were five composite restorations on the teeth for a total value of about $1600. None were crowns, 3/4 crowns, nor were crowns indicated. To me, it was a clear case of fraud.

Fraud is fairly difficult to prove: there are three factors. First, there must be financial damage. In this case $2400 cost difference between treatment rendered vs. the treatment charged. Second, the dentist must have knowledge of the act and intent. If a staff member mischarged a patient, or the dentist made a simple mistake, it is not fraud. In this case the dentist admitted that he did know. Third, there has to be a pattern. In this case we showed some other restorations had been similarly billed several years earlier. The case was sent to our disciplinary board. They returned it. One of the board members always submitted his composite fillings this way because there was at one time no code for composite restorations and it was the only way he could get paid for them. At the time, appropriate codes existed and were not used because insurance companies would not pay for the composite restorations but would pay for gold crowns. How silly of me to think this was inappropriate treatment.

A dentist should report bad treatment

As an insurance consultant, I occasionally see cases of bad treatment. This treatment is well beyond the overtreatment I see on a regular basis. Over the years we have identified several offices that seem to have an unusually high incidence of such work. I sent about 20 cases to our Quality Assurance Commission. All came from 5 or 6 offices. These cases had been reviewed by 10 senior dentists, most of whom taught full or part time at the dental school. To the person they were appalled at the treatment. Surely, the board would take a look. If nothing else, they could go to the office and do a random audit of charts. What was their conclusion? Since the patient did not file the complaint, they would not review the cases.

Who is better able to assess the quality of care, the patient or 10 respected dentists?

A clear case of fraud

Is it a matter of degree or the amount of money involved? Let's look at the case of two young men right out of school. They were movers. They wanted to be successful. After a year in separate practices they joined forces in a clinic. They advertised in phone books, on buses, and billboards, and in a short time had a very busy, successful practice. They took welfare patients. Folks on welfare have a very difficult time finding dentists to do their care because the state's payments often are below what it costs to do the treatment before the dentist gets paid. In spite of this, the practice of our two young dentists became primarily welfare. They provided a needed service and advertised it well. Their practice grew beyond their wildest dreams. How did they work within a system with such low fees? It was simple: everyone that walked into the office got bite guards. This was a way to inflate fees. I suspect even the mailman who delivered the mail probably was fitted for one. There are those who think almost everyone needs a bite guard to sleep in and they certainly fill this possible need. However, they were financially successful beyond anyone's dream. How could this be? They had a simple technique. Do every tooth that even hinted of decay, but charge for fillings on two or three teeth for every one you treated.

They eventually were found out. It was estimated that they had defrauded the state for over a million dollars. No one really knows how much it was. Now, surely this met the criteria of fraud. They were convicted and fined $400,000. They practiced as a corporation. The corporation lost its ability to serve as a dental company. Both were given jail time, but were allowed to do community service in lieu of actual jail time. They were both back in practice within 6 months They had taken continuing education courses during the three months they could not practice and worked in free clinics. For this, one was awarded a Fellowship in the Academy of General Dentistry and the other was nominated for a Jefferson Award that was announced in the local newspaper. Talk about taking lemons and making lemonade.

Since this first brush with the licensing board, one has gone on to more sanctions by the board, eventually losing his license.

Death

Surely, you'd think, death would cause some stern action. Not necessarily so. There was a case a few years ago where a 51-year-old patient died after oral surgery to place some implants. The case was very sad. I first learned of it when a friend, who is an anesthesiologist, called me to see what the standard was for monitoring general anesthesia by dentists. He described a case where the patient had a blood pressure taken prior to the start of treatment and was given multiple drugs several times, eventually leading to her having a cardiac arrest.

The surgeon at this point started breathing for her but never started the chest compression of CPR. They did call the paramedics who managed to get the patient's heart restarted. The paramedics got a blood pressure measurement after restarting the patient's heart. This was the first measurement of her blood pressure since before the case was started.

A local surgeon testified that she had a bounding pulse and with that you did not need to take blood pressures. In my anesthesia residency, I took blood pressures at least every 5 minutes, more often if there were changes. Other monitors were available but not used by this surgeon. The patient passed away several days later in the hospital. The only question is how she lived as long as she did, considering the variety and amounts of drugs that were administered. Even so, she might have lived had she been monitored and if her cardiac arrest had been noticed earlier and if proper CPR had been preformed.

All this went to the disciplinary board, which has the ultimate authority over our license. They decided it was an unfortunate outcome and could not be considered reason to pull a license, because they did not have a regulation requiring monitoring patents under general anesthesia. They did call a committee to review the lack of regulations.

The disciplinary board decided the dentist had exceeded the standard of care but could be a little better at record keeping. He distributed the letter from the board to all his referring doctors as vindication that he had not done anything wrong. It was just an unfortunate outcome.

In defense of the board, the oral surgery community had closed ranks and testified to the board that everything that had been done was standard care. The board gave the surgeon's testimony more weight than the medical anesthesiologist who was very critical of the case.

Several months later, one of the surgeons got up in a meeting that was reviewing the case and stated that we do not have to be perfect. CPR is comprised of three things: establishing an airway, breathing for the patient, and chest compression. He did two out of three. We do not have to be perfect.

The dentist lost another patient a few years later. There were no sanctions in this death either.

Public access to records

The Dental Disciplinary Board used to print the

names and a brief description of the incident that led to the sanctioning of a dentist. These records of completed cases are public. It should be possible to ask the board for a report of transgressions of your dentist. However, there were two dentists in our state with the same first and last names. One was sanctioned by the board. The other just happened to be president of our state dental association. It was the last time reports of dentists were published in our dental journals.

You can find the reports of cases where there was legal action on the state's website. These are public record. If there was a complaint that did not result in a formal legal action, you can get these records because they too are public; however, you must ask for the specific dentist and a specific treatment and be willing to pay for the state's cost for copying the records of the board meeting for the specific incident. The ability and ease of getting records vary from state to state.

National Practitioner Database

How about the national practitioner database? If a dentist or physician is sanctioned by a disciplinary board, dental association, loses a malpractice suit, or even refunds fees for a procedure, this is turned in to the National Practitioner Database, the record or a report of the incident is to be forwarded to this national repository of problems. This has actually led to ending some peer review panels as if the dental association sanctioned one of their own, it would require a report. If they did not have a review process then no report would be generated.

While the concept of such a database sounds good, it has eliminated some of the mechanisms a patient could use when they felt they had been mistreated. You would expect that you could go to this database and find out if a potential doctor has a record of problems. In fact, it is almost impossible for an individual to get access to this information. Only hospitals, peer review organizations, licensing boards, and similar bodies can get reports from the database.

As you may have guessed, I had about given up on our Dental Quality Assurance Commission. I decided it was unfair to be critical if I did not try to make changes. It took 8 years but I got appointed to the Commission and have managed to help start the process of change. I cooperated with an investigation by one of our newspapers. I was criticized by other board members for talking and was accused of giving out patients' names. I had been unable to get the names. The reporter was truly remarkable in her research of the cases. Her fair, detailed, and critical reporting of the cases has nudged the commission into making changes.

Largely because I did these reviews, I am being challenged. I may be removed from the board for this. Also cited was the fact that I teach continuing education courses, do research, publish research papers, and do insurance reviews. I was told by the state that this is like the military, you have to obey the orders of the chairman and the state supervisor. This is strange. I thought I was appointed because of all my activities and I was to vote my conscience.

The system is very slow. All board meetings are public except when a case is being deliberated. Once a decision is made, that decision becomes public record. All changes to regulations must be done in public meeting after publishing the topic of the meeting, then the proposed changes, then accepting public input, and finally publishing that a final vote will be taken. All of this will take at least six months for simple changes and over a year for significant changes. Public access is very important but it makes it very difficult to respond to needs for change in a timely manner.

Insurance reviews

There is one somewhat effective mechanism of review for some patients. That is the insurance review. For the more expensive dental procedures that are covered by insurance companies or welfare trust, there is a review process to assess the need for the treatment, its appropriateness, and whether the treatment is covered by the plan.

Those of us who do insurance reviews get a lot of bad comments. Many dentists believe we are paid by the number of cases we deny. Nothing could be farther from the truth. We decide if a treatment is covered by the plan and then if it is appropriate treatment.

On a personal basis, I have been sworn at by dentists, dental assistants, and patients. I was once referred to as an insurance whore. My response was, "but you should see me in my net stocking, leather skirt, and low cut blouse." Some treatments that we do not approve for payment are simply not covered under the insurance policy. Others fail the test because there are less costly alternatives that are appropriate, and a few fail because the prognosis of such treatment is very poor. Now and again, a case comes my way that I am very proud of.

This patient was abandoned

A 30 year old woman went to a dentist. She had very crowded front teeth. From the x-rays I'd say she probably had an unpleasant smile. She and her husband were both members of the same union. This union has a very good plan that even covers some implants. However, if more than three teeth are missing in one arch, upper or lower, the plan will not pay to have them replaced with implants, but will pay for a partial denture.

The dentist told the patient that between her and her husband's insurance they would pay 100% for removing her 4 front teeth, placing 4 implants and then 4 porcelain crowns. He promised her a beautiful smile by Christmas. He removed the teeth, placed the implants and eventually placed temporary crowns on the implants. The temporaries did not look much like teeth and were way too white. At this point the dentist sent in an insurance form to get paid for the implants.

The review came to me and was denied because there were 4 missing teeth—the trust did not cover 4 implants; they would redirect treatment to a partial denture in such a case. Her bill from the dentist for 4 implants and crowns would be a little over $10,000; her coverage was $500, which is 50% of the cost of a partial denture. Her husband had been laid off and no longer had insurance. Once it was clear that the patient did not have coverage, the dentist refused to see her.

The patient appealed her coverage to the Union Trust. It was a sad case. She clearly did not have benefits for the treatment, much less the treatment that was left to do. She could not afford to pay for the treatment that had been started. The trust members listened to all of this and adjourned to decide what they should do. They decided they had latitude enough to cover the implants and crowns at their normal rate. This would give her $8000 of coverage rather than $500 that was actually prescribed by the plan. That would still leave her owing $2000, which she clearly could not afford. The trust members looked at me. I asked if I could try to make a deal with the dentist. They agreed.

I was on the phone for about 30 minutes. The conversation went something like this:

I started by explaining that I had been authorized to offer him $8000 if this case was completed by Christmas and he excused the remaining $2000 cost.

This is between the patient and her insurance company, he said. He would just sue her.

"You do not seem to understand," I explained patiently. "I can get you $8000 instead of the $500 that is now scheduled to be paid to you."

He would not hear of it. He would sue, and take her house and car.

I tried to reason with him. "She has no house and you would not want her car." I did not know this but a bluff was in order. "However, the trust will pay $8000 rather than $500 that is actually covered if you excuse the unpaid $2000."

"I will just take her to court for the rest", he repeated stubbornly.

I decided the time for niceties was over. "You seem to be a slow learner," I said. "You have abandoned her. A, I will get her to a sleazy attorney and you will be sued and lose about $30,000 or $40,000, maybe much more that that, but will receive $500 or B, you can get paid $8000 if you finish the case by Christmas and excuse the remaining $2000. Which do you want A or B?"

He finally got it. "Well," he admitted slowly, "if you put it that way I guess I will accept the $8,000." The trust was happy with my negotiating skills and one of supervisors who is in the office next to mine said, "The next time I negotiate a raise you are coming with me." The patient will never know what I did for her but it sure left me with a good feeling.

Each State will have different criteria for their Board or Commission. In general:

- do not attempt to take fee disputes.
- do not attempt to take personality complaints.

Go to the state board or commission if:
- you feel your work was defective.
- you felt there were some sexual improprieties.
- you feel you were assaulted or abused.

Realize that some boards are not very aggressive. As we have seen, sometimes the state will pressure the commission members to accept compromise or the state bureaucrats may simply refuse to take action. So start with peer review and go on to the licensing board if you feel you were wronged. Realize that you probably will not be able to sue short of very severe damage to nerves, jaws, or serious infections. Most tooth problems are simply not worth enough to justify an attorney taking your case on a contingency.

So who looks out for you?

So who looks out for you, the patient? The answer is you do. It is the goal of this book to give you enough information to ask the good questions, know what procedures to be suspicious of, and have enough information to make rational decisions.

What happens if I do nothing and how long will that take?

If you do not want to get into all the details, there are two simple things you can do: always ask what happens if instead of the recommended treatment you do nothing, and how long will it take to happen.

Nothing is sometimes the best treatment. Remember, you are never wrong going for a second opinion. Your insurance or trust might even provide for this. They might be willing to provide this service at no cost or might even suggest the names of appropriate dentists to do such a review. The most it will cost you is about 20% of the cost of a single crown and can save you hundreds if not thousands of dollars.

Remember, there is little we do as dentists that is as good as what you originally had. Now, if you have decay, gum disease, or infection, you might have no options other than treatment. But remember, the decision is yours as to what treatment you have done. It is your mouth and your wallet.

Check out your dentist

You should check out your dentist by doing a web search using the name of the state you are in, Dental Board, or dental disciplinary board or Dental Quality Assurance commission, or simply call your state dental licensing board and ask for the record of the dentist you are interested in. Most states have web pages where you can search for the record of any licensed dentist.

For the full list of state dental licensing boards, visit this Web page: http://www.dentalwatch. org/org/boards.html

You check out a used car before you purchase it, but you pick a physician or dentist on the recommendation of a friend or because of their advertising. It does not make a lot of sense.

II. Who is your dentist?

HERMAN® by Jim Unger

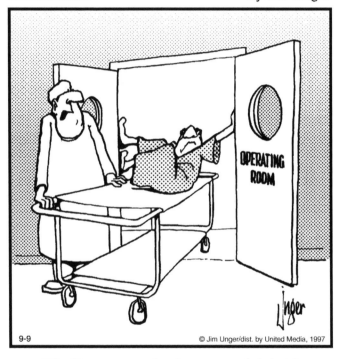

9-9 © Jim Unger/dist. by United Media, 1997

**"Er, Doc ... can he have a quick look
at your diploma?"**

3. Credentialing

Games boys play

There is a game little boys play in country towns. They gather out behind the barn and see who can pee the highest up the wall. The winner pees on his head. Professionals play a similar game. They get together socially and soon are comparing degrees.

I have a DDS
I have an MD
I have a DDS MD
I have a DDS MD PhD
I got my PhD at the University of Washington
I got my PhD at the Stanford University
I got my PhD at Harvard

He wins, and everyone hates him.

A friend of mine met a dentist socially. In a short conversation she was told he had retired, had a new wife, and thus had to go back to practicing and that he graduated first in his dental class at UCLA. She met a grandfather at a park playing with his grandchild. She began talking to his wife who explained he was a recently retired physician who was enjoying his grandchildren. After the physician and his wife left the park, another mom asked my friend if she knew who that was. She did not have a clue. It turned out he was one of the prime cancer researchers in the country. Those who have it do not have to advertise.

Buyer beware

There was a time when advertising was a no-no in medicine and dentistry. That all changed about 25 years ago when it was declared restraint of trade to restrict advertising. The best advice is buyer beware. What can you believe? There are regulations about false advertising that help a bit. You can not claim to be a specialist if you are not a specialist. Some areas of dentistry should have specialty status, but so far it has been blocked. Anesthesiology and implants are two specialties that would make sense. The surgery community has blocked any attempt at recognizing these two areas.

> *When I was in the military we had battalion meetings every week of all the officers. The commanding officer started around the room. Mr. Smith, do you have anything? Mr. Jones, do you have anything? Mr. Bliss, do you have anything? Mr. Quarnstrom, do you have anything. Dr. Star, do ... Sitting on a beachhead in a war zone makes you a little crazy. Crazy is the norm. This bugged me to no end. One day I wrote an official letter from the Dental Officer to the Commanding Officer. I quoted Navy regulations that stated a dentist should be referred to as Dr. until he made Commander at which time either title was appropriate. I was doctored after that but I paid big time by getting every garbage job the CO could come up with. I learned a valuable lesson at an early stage of my career. You earn your title every day from the people you care for. You cannot just demand respect.*

What do the initials mean?

Many practitioners try to look like specialists by using designations of awards they have received. It is against the ethics of most organizations to let dentists report their fellowships in advertising except for letter heads and possibly business cards and in professional publications. To an extent this is unfortunate.

To decide what designations are significant and what are not is a minefield we will attempt to help you navigate.

Academy of General Dentistry

The Academy of General Dentistry had Fellowship and Mastership awards. The Fellowship, FAGD, indicates a dentist took a rather extensive test on all aspects of dentistry and has 500 hours of continuing education on clinical topics. There also is a requirement of yearly continuing education. The mastership program, MAGD, includes another 500 hours with most being hands-on clinical courses in a variety of dental areas. Both indicate dentists who have continued their learning but they cannot tell patients. This makes little sense. It would encourage other dentists to do the same. Does this guarantee competency? No, but it is an indication.

Anesthesia and other initials

The American Dental Society of Anesthesiology has a fellowship, FADSA, program that used to require a full year of anesthesia training. In the past, they have granted a few fellowships to dentists with as little as a 3-month training program in anesthesia. This has now been abandoned so you do not know what it really certifies. There is an American Society of Dental Anesthesiology that requires a full 2 year residency in anesthesia, 1 year for us old folks who were grandfathered in, because 2 year programs did not exist 30 years ago. There are also fellowships associated with other accomplishments in dental leadership or other dental accomplishment. These include the Fellow of the International College of Dentistry, FICD, that is offered to less than 5% of dentists each year and the Fellow in the American College of Dentistry, FACD, that is awarded to about 1 or 2% of dentists each year, again for their accomplishments.

The me too organizations and plaques

There are other organizations that grant fellowships, masterships, and diplomates. Some are a sign of accomplishments; others are more a matter of attending a few classes and spending some, to a lot, of money for the certificate. Every now and again there will be a brochure that states "I have been chosen as one of America's most outstanding dentists and I can have a plaque or award for only $350 or more depending on the size of the plaque and the more impressive mounting." I had to laugh when a neurologist was proudly interviewed by a TV station standing in front of his outstanding certificate. If only patients knew what they stood for. It is a great way to unload plaques when a manufacturer has a surplus or a rather inventive way to start a certificate business.

Seattle's best dentists, or are they?

Next we have the magazines reporting on a city's best restaurants, hotels, chefs, physicians, dentists, etc. Seattle has just such a magazine. Each year the most outstanding dentists are listed. If you want some fun, look up the nominees on your state's licensing board. Our most outstanding had been disciplined for prescribing drugs beyond his license including narcotics for himself. Another had two patients die in his office and was featured in a three part exposure in one of the daily newspapers a few months before he was named by the Seattle magazine as one of the best. Some of those named really are the cream of the crop. Others take out large multi-page ads in the magazine. I am sure that is not why they were named. It sort of makes you wonder, however.

Brochures in the supermarket

Ever wonder why dentists put glossy brochures in the super markets of upscale neighborhoods? These are very expensive to have designed, photographed, printed and they pay to have them in the grocery store. Why do they do it? Because it works. People look at these and do not see a skillful advertiser, they think they guarantee quality. There is no guarantee. It almost seems that those in the upscale wealthy neighborhoods are more vulnerable than others. You would not expect that they got to their exalted neighborhoods because they were very gullible.

TV stations experts

I was offered the chance to be featured on the web site of one of our local TV stations as one of the experts. At last someone was recognizing my genius. I soon discovered that my genius was appreciated but only if I agreed to pay $3700 a month for the privilege. I decided my ego would have to get along without that citation. I can only guess what it costs one of our local dentists to have two or three ads an evening during prime time.

Be wary of superiority claims

What can you believe about those ads? The dentist can afford to pay for them because you must pay up front to be featured. They must work as they are very costly or the dentists are as gullible as the patients who believe them. I think informational ads make sense, come to us because we do fillings, crowns, extractions, bridges, dentures, use nitrous oxide or sedation. These are factual about what an office does. As soon as the ad suggests that the dentist is an expert in some aspect of dentistry, is one of the city's best dentists, was named the most outstanding dentist by a magazine or TV, is in the top 5% of dentists because they purchased a plaque, or attended an institute, be very wary.

Do not be fooled

It might be worth asking for a resume or Curriculum Vitae. Not all dentists will have a CV or resume. If they can produce it quickly (do not give them 4 days to phony up one), have it printed off a computer, copied off a copy machine, it may be valid. It will tend to indicate that they have spoken to a dental group and had to prepare one. This may be a good sign.

Abraham Lincoln said you can fool some of the people all of the time, and all of the people some of the time, but you cannot fool all of the people all of the time. But you do not have to fool all of them all the time to be successful advertising. Be very wary of advertising claims.

You are far better off asking friends and acquaintances about their dentists. Ask what they like or do not like. What sort of procedures they have had done. Be particularly suspicious if you live in an upscale neighborhood.

4. Getting to Know Your Dentist

Choosing the right dentist is a very personal decision. We all make decisions based upon our own personalities and experiences. This chapter will help you make the decision that is right for you.

Dentistry is a medical profession. It provides an important service and it is a business. This business can be as lucrative as the dentists decide they want it to be based upon their management of their office and the treatment decisions they make in your mouth.

Dental practitioners operate in a world of mixed messages. The dentist is supposed to be your health advocate, and yet their economic livelihood depends on the amount of work they do in your mouth. Keep this in mind as you make your decisions.

Our aim is to help you understand the differences in care, training, and management in the care of your mouth.

Dental training

Dentists and their staff have varying degrees of training and standards of care. It is smart to examine the qualifications of the people who are taking care of your health. This sounds obvious, and yet most people do not do this. In fact, most people do not ask questions about the training and qualifications of medical health practitioners and their staff. But a well-trained and competent medical practitioner will be proud to tell you about themselves. A simple call to the front desk asking about the training of the dentist and their staff is easy to make. Go ahead, ask.

Ask about your dentist's qualifications

Every dentist must be licensed. However, dentists that earned fellowships, have taken advanced classes and have extra qualifications often offer a higher standard of care. The cost of the treatment is usually the same, so why not use a dentist who is interested enough in what they are doing to take some continuing education, CE?

Fellowship or Mastership in the Academy of General Dentistry guarantees 500 and 1,000 hours of CE, and a tough all-day test. Other certification may not be as difficult to achieve. Still others will guarantee only that the dentist knows how to market dentistry.

The basics

A simple measure of quality care starts with a complete exam of your teeth, your gums, your tongue, and other soft tissues of your mouth. Often it will include a palpation of the head and neck. This should not go below the clavicle, collar-bone. This exam must be done by a dentist.

The dental assistant

Some states require the dental assistants to have training and credentials, and others do not. If you move to a state that does not require specific training, you might notice the difference in the procedures done by assistants. Usually x-rays will be taken by the dental assistant. They may take impressions for study models.

The dental hygienist

A dental hygienist might be the person that does your cleanings. Assistants are not allowed to clean teeth. They are allowed by some states to polish teeth after a dentist or hygienist has removed the hard deposits, calculus, or tartar. If an assistant is doing the cleaning, you want to find a different place for care. All states require a dental hygienist to have at least a two-year hygiene course. Some require two years of pre-hygiene courses to be admitted to a hygiene program.

Ethics and philosophy

When starting a new dental care relationship, you will want to align your care team with your personal style. A dentist who is impatient with questions may not be someone you want as a provider if you are someone who likes to be informed. A practitioner who focuses exclusively on cosmetics may not be the person you want taking care of your teeth if your sole objective is disease prevention. You will not care if the dentist received the aesthetic dentist award with veneers and bleaching if that is not what you are after. As you age, your needs will change. A young mouth needs prevention rather than restoration. During middle age you may need someone who is monitoring gum disease and the beginning of teeth preservation.

A simple rule of thumb is to trust your instincts and match yourself with someone who has a treatment philosophy that is consistent with your objectives. If you visit a dentist and it doesn't feel right, trust yourself.

Young vs. old dentists

Young dentists are enthusiastic and up to date in their training. They do not have the years of experience, but they have just been shown how to use the new materials with the most up to date equipment. The schools are 10 years behind new technology. This is not all good or bad. The recent grad has just enough knowledge to not be too dangerous. There is a balance of experience that may cause a more experienced dentist to be able to make a better judgment in a complex case. Sometimes, professionals learn tricks that benefit the patient directly.

An example of this was an acquaintance whose special needs child would not open his mouth, which made an exam impossible. The young dentist had the patient come back three times with no luck. The child simply would not let the cleaning take place. This had an economic cost because there were three treatment blocks on the schedule and booked staff time. The patient's mother mentioned this experience to a dentist who had practiced for twenty-five years. The older dentist suggested a dose of benadryl just before the appointment. The mother tried this with great success, resulting in a terrific cleaning experience, and six months later the child went through his follow up without any problem. The young dentist found this to be a hugely helpful change in his treatment plan and has since adopted this standard with fearful pediatric patients.

Another example of differences in approaches to dental care is a senior dentist and a new associate. The patients who need appliance work always go to the senior dentist because he tinkers with their appliance and fixes it. He regards this as part of his job. The young dentist takes an impression and orders a new one, resulting in more billable care and a higher profit for him. The patients in this practice are noticing this and spreading the word. The senior dentist who only works two days a week has a full patient load with a waiting list and the associate has open time. The number of patients in the practice is eroding.

Emergency care

Some dentists charge a consulting fee for returning phone calls. An after hours call is billed out. Others do not charge for these after-hours consultations. Some offices have no emergency coverage. Others have a plan for care every day of the week and evenings if necessary, 24/7. Check out the details before you need the service. It might mean the difference between preserving a tooth, or being pain free. This might not seem important to you until you have been up all night with a problem.

Appointments

Some dentists will always be on time. If you have a 10:15 appointment, the dentist will walk into the treatment room at 10:15. Others are never on time. Occasional delays are inevitable, but expecting patients to always wait shows a lack of respect for the patient. Cancellations are also a matter of practice management. It really is not fair to a dentist to not show for an appointment. Many offices will call and remind you of your appointment. Some charge for missed appointments.

Marketing

Some dentists are slick. They have beautiful offices, great plants, and they offer coffee, tea, and beverages. When you are a new patient, there is a certain amount of sales on the part of the practice. On average a dentist retains close to 100% of their new patients if they are caring and do not oversell. It is worth their time to woo you and to keep you. Some offer incentives for referring new patients. This can include free bleaching kits, services, gift certificates, concert tickets, and even as trite as it sounds, wine and roses. I am suspicious of these approaches. It seems to me that patient satisfaction is the best form of advertisement. Besides, who do you think pays for all this?

Different parts of the country have different standards for this sort of marketing. Some areas offer incentives for joining a practice: a free set of x-rays, a bleach kit, a toothbrush, and a free exam. There is more competition in some areas than there is in others. Just keep your eyes open.

Check your dentist's record

Each state has a state licensing board. It never hurts to check on the status of your health practitioner to see if there have been any major infractions and corrections during the time they have practiced. Once again, information is power.

Questions to ask as you join a dental practice

- What are the academic qualifications of your dentist?
- How many continuing education hours do they have?
- How long have they been practicing?
- What is the emergency coverage for the office?
- What are the payment and insurance policies?
- How hard is it to get an appointment when you have an emergent problem?

- Does the doctor stand behind his or her work?
- How much emphasis does the care team give to medical history?
- If using sedation, what qualifications does the dentist have?
- Are their emergency procedures up to date?
- Is there a prevention program for decay and gum disease?
- Is the office clean?
- Is the office staff pleasant?
- Does the care team answer your questions and present you with options?
- Does the hygienist receive an economic incentive for selling certain procedures?
- Will the office remind you and schedule hygiene or is it your responsibility?

5. Referrals

Sir, if I cannot put my hand in your mouth, I will have to refer you to a specialist.

It is OK for me to refer you, if you need a service I cannot provide.

It is OK for you to request a referral at any time.

When is a referral necessary?

A referral is in order whenever a patient requests one. It is never wrong to ask for a second opinion. You are never wrong to tell your general dentist you would like to see a specialist for a procedure. If you get any resistance from your dentist, you may be going to the wrong dentist.

What can general dentists do?

A general dentist can do anything they are qualified to do. That includes peridodontal treatments, root canals, orthodontics, and surgery. The basics of all these are learned in school. That is why they call it "practice." If I want to learn about a new area, I will read journals, books, and take classes. I may join a study club that meets on a monthly basis with an expert in that area.

I learned surgery on a beachhead in Vietnam. I was right out of dental school and had done under 20 extractions. I found myself responsible for a battalion of young men. Their average age was about 22. One of their major problems was their impacted and infected wisdom teeth, 3rd molars.

I had never done an extraction of an impacted tooth before. There was no one I could refer these patients to. Many would come to me with potentially serious infections. I often would treat the patients with an assistant holding open the surgery book so I would know what to do next. I had a very primitive office, no suction, no water or air syringe. What I did have was several large ear syringes to provide suction, air, and water. I had the ability to think my way around these problems.

I learned a lot of surgery that year. I did extractions that I will now refer out to surgeons because I think they can do a better job if there are complications. I did not have that option in Vietnam. I was "the man," inexperienced as I was. Within a year there were oral surgeons at Chu Lai. By then I was back in the US. My year in Vietnam was a great learning experience and because of it I do 80% of the surgery needed by my patients. As I have said, that is why it is referred to as "a dental practice."

I am competent to do most extractions. I am competent to handle the complication of the procedures that I do. When I see a need that has even a small chance of a complication I am not comfortable with, I will refer to a specialist.

How do I choose a specialist?

I want my patients to be comfortable with the specialist I refer them to. Therefore, I am careful to check out a few things. First, I look at their credentials. Where did they take their training? Do they teach? Do they write? Are they nice people who will relate to my patients?

I did a 10 Saturday "mini residency" in endodontics, root canals. There were 7 instructors. One was head of endodontics at the local dental school but did no clinical practice—can't use him. Three were from out of town—too far to drive. Two were very competent but very brisk, did not explain well, and were snobs. Anyone can go to a jerk, but I will not refer to them unless they are clearly superior to others and I will warn the patient of what to expect. The last was one of the kindest most concerned people I had ever met. In addition he was one of the most competent. Needless to say he's the one I refer my patients to for all those root canals I cannot do.

He got very busy very fast, so he brought in a new man. I knew the new fellow could not be as nice. He may, in fact, be even nicer. Within a few years they both were booked out 2 months. They brought in a woman endodontist. She may be the nicest of the bunch.

I never worry when I refer to them. I always get glowing reports back from my patients. My only concern is three people cannot be this nice 24/7. They must get into their autos to go home and swear the whole way home. Maybe they get home, put on boxing gloves and hit a bag to get rid of frustrations. They must have some form of release because some of what they do is very stressful and very demanding. I do not send them the easy root canals.

I will almost always give you a choice of two or three specialists

I will also describe each in some detail. Maybe you want to go to a woman (or a man). Maybe you want to go to someone close to your home. Maybe you are a minority and are more comfortable with someone of your own race. Maybe you want a role model for your children. See, women can be orthodontists, see African-Americans can be orthodontists. Maybe you want to go to someone who teaches part time at the dental school.

There are some procedures that are so complex that you want to be in the hands of someone who does a lot of these. In this case I may refer you only to the person I know who is superior to all others in the area. I will tell you why I refer only to this person for this procedure.

I will not send you to someone I think is incompetent. There is an oral surgeon in our town who has had two people die of anesthesia complications. I have no problem telling people not to go to that office. I will not send you to jerks. I will not send you to someone who does not communicate back to me as to what they did, what to expect, what I have to worry about. I will not refer you to someone I do not know.

I will stop referring to anyone who crosses any line or does anything that I think is inappropriate.

I had referred to a surgeon for years, probably 2 or 3 patients a week. I sent the boyfriend of my assistant to him for 4 impacted wisdom teeth, 3rd molars. Three were very difficult. He charged a fair fee for these three. One was a gimme, it was so easy, it could have fallen out in his hand. He charged for a surgical extraction. It was a very simple extraction. This bounced his fee about $100. I called and asked him why. He said," I am very upset you are questioning me." I said, "I am very distressed I have to make this call."

I never referred to him again. This cost him about $15,000 to $20,000 a week in lost referrals. I hope the $100 upgraded fee was worth it.

I had another surgeon who I used after I quit the one above. I had used him for about 15 years. I sent a 10 year old to have a bump removed from his lip. I could have done it but the child needed to be sedated, because he was frightened. The surgeon must have been behind as he tried to shame the child into letting him do it with local anesthesia. It was a bad scene and nothing got done. The child's parents were mad as hell. That just cost him $20,000 a week. I am now referring to a different surgeon.

What I do not like about some specialists

Now and again I will attend a course put on by a specialist who makes statements such as, "If you do not refer all your periodontal patients to me, you are supervising their neglect and I will have to serve with the prosecution if they have a problem." I call this the, "I walk on water" syndrome. I know they are good or I would not go to their course, but I want someone who can relate to the average patients. I never refer to such specialists. "It is nice to be smart, but it is smarter to be nice."

I have several specialists who have encouraged me to do root canals, surgery, and periodontal treatments. If I have a problem, they are happy to see the patient. I cannot count the number of times I have opened into a root canal and been unable to find all the canals. Many times the canals get smaller with age, sometimes to the extent that they are not visible even with a microscope. I get the patient out of pain but I cannot do the root canal. The specialists gladly accept these patients. I have also broken off roots of teeth that I was extracting and I simply could not get the root. They were happy to see the patient and recover the root. Thankfully, this doesn't happen very often; in the case of the root fractures, there have been 3 times in 30 years. Not being able to find a canal happens about once a month.

Why not always go to a specialist?

You can always see a specialist if you so choose. That is your option. There are patients who should always go to specialists because they need bragging rights among their friends. They need to be able to say they drove 50 miles because Dr. X is so good. They need to be able to say they paid three times what you did to get their root canal done. They need to say their specialist was so smart they would not even talk to them.

Many general dentists are capable of doing much of what specialists do. I do around 300 root canals a year and probably 500 extractions. I charge less than a specialist. I can do this because I do the easy and moderately difficult cases. I send the specialists the impossible ones. I can do this because I already know you, I do not have to make a separate appointment to see what you need and get to know you.

Sometimes the specialist has specialized equipment that is costly so they can do more difficult procedures. They can charge more as specialists because they have had 3 or 4 extra years of training, the insurance companies will pay them more, and they can demand higher fees because they are specialists.

It is always your choice of going to a specialist

Before you decide who will do a procedure for you, ask your dentist the following questions: How many of these have you done? Are you comfortable doing them? What special training have you taken? What will it cost if you do it? About what will it cost if I go to the specialist? Why are you sending me to the specialist? They should be willing and able to answer all these questions. My personal feeling is specialists are there to do the difficult procedures. I can keep the cost down by doing the less complex procedures.

HERMAN®

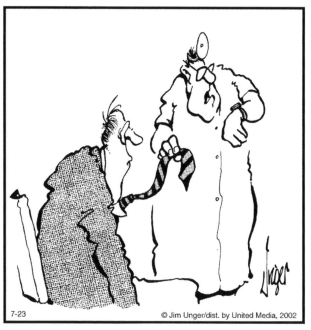

"Your pulse is very, very weak!"

6. Your medical history:
Let's get acquainted

One of my patients said the following:

I expected your staff to ask my name.
I expected them to ask for my address.
I expected them to ask about my insurance.
I was surprised at the medical history I had to fill out.
You know more about me than my doctor or my wife.
I was concerned, however, when your staff asked for my next-of- kin.
He was just joking about the next-of-kin.

Medical history

When you visit your dentist for the first time, they will ask you to fill out a medical history form. It might seem boring and inconsequential to you, but all those details are actually extremely important and might save your life one day.

Make sure they review the form

Be sure your dentist takes a look at the medical history form you have so carefully filled out. Ask them if they have any questions or need more information. I always initial and date the form as proof I have reviewed it. I also ask you to review it every year and update any changes, and we both sign the form at that time.

The dentist needs to know about your medical problems

In general, your dentist needs to know about any diseases you have, any drugs you are taking, and any bad habits, such as smoking, bulimia, or dietary issues. And yes, it does mean any recreational drugs. It is also very important to reveal any medical conditions. I have included the form I use to record a medical history. This is a starting place. If a patient answers yes to any question I often ask them follow up questions so I know all I need to know to safely treat them. I may even contact their physician to ask for more details. Do I really need to know all that stuff? In a word, "Yes!"

For example, if you report you have had a heart attack. I will want to know more details. How long ago was that? Have you had a second or third attack? What treatments did they do for you? Did they use clot busters, a stent, a balloon dilation? About every 4 years I will find someone who is sick enough I think they should be treated in a hospital. What medications do you take? Does it restrict what you can do?

If they use a less complete form, use ours

Copy our form, fill it out, and give it to your dentist if they do not have a similar form. You want them to know all about your medical problems even if they do not ask. I would start to be a little suspicious if they do not collect this information. It would make me wonder: What else do they not do that they should?

The good news about going to the dentist is it is very rare to see a life threatening complication, particularly if you are not getting IV sedation or general anesthesia. Local anesthesia is very safe. We no longer use Novocain, procaine. We have not used Novocain for at least 40 years, but local anesthetics are commonly referred to by patients as Novocain. We have much more potent and safer drugs today.

The bad news is that because we rarely see medical emergencies we do not get much practice handling emergency events (not that we really want the opportunity to practice on you). If I have a patient faint, it has been a bad year. We practice what we will do in emergencies; but, at best, we depend on paramedic backup for serious problems. We will never be as capable as the EMT folks or the hospital emergency department who see serious emergencies every shift. For this reason we need your help before an emergency situation arises. Tell us about yourself so we know what to do when something goes wrong.

Tobacco use (Smoking and smokeless)

We all know how dangerous tobacco is. In addition to screwing up your heart, lungs, blood vessels, kidneys, eyes etc., smoking stains your teeth. That is not a major problem, as we can clean off these stains, it just means your cleaning costs more. However, if you smoke, it is very detrimental to your gum tissue. If you have the two bad genes we will talk about and you smoke, you have a much greater chance of having sever,e refractory to treatment, gum disease. You will probably start losing teeth in your 30s if you have this defect and smoke.

Smokeless tobacco is also bad

You will see the same if you "chew". The little pinch between your gums and teeth not only makes your breath smell like a spittoon from a grade B cowboy movie, but also causes tissue changes that can and do lead to oral cancer. It is not uncommon to see young men and sometimes women with a white patch on their gums. This is a thickening of the tissue that results from the irritation to the chemical in tobacco. One rather well publicized case was a professional baseball Player who lost half his jaw. He goes around talking to youth about the terrible problem that was caused by chewing.

I had a young patient who chewed. I was on his case like bugs on poop. Every 6 months we played the game of "Can you tell where I am putting the tobacco now?" This went on for about 3 years. Once he came in and said, "I bet you cannot find the place today." I searched high and low, back and forward, under the tongue, in the cheeks. On the back of his tongue. He had me stumped, I could not find the whitish patch. I said, "OK where are you putting it?", He said, "You can't find it?" I said, "no." He said, "that is because I quit. My new girlfriend would not kiss me if I kept chewing. She said my mouth tasted terrible." YES! She had success where I had failed. Go girls.

Smoking cigars and pipes can also cause terrible tissue reactions. They can turn the tongue black because of the tars in tobacco. One of the worst things you can do is sit down with a glass of strong liquor and a cigar. The alcohol bares the surface of the oral tissues and the cigar's chemicals have direct access to these tissues. Even for the nonsmoker or occasional smoker this can have devastating effects.

Reverse smoking is the worst

Every now and again I find a reverse smoker, or someone who puts the lit end of the cigarette in their mouth. This is probably the worst form of smoking. I have seen the top of mouths, the palate, look like cottage cheese from this insult. I also had one elderly patient whose denture was burned from the heat of the lit end of the cigarette.

If you smoke, quit. If you failed last time, try again. That previous time was only a rehearsal for this time that is going to work. I quit after 15 years. It was one of the most difficult things I ever did. I have been smokeless for 15 years. It took 10 years to get rid of the urge. I probably quit 10 times before I got it right and it lasted. If you do not smoke, do not start. If you smoke, quit, quit, quit, and quit. One of the times it will be for good. *There is nothing worse than a reformed smoker.*

Dietary habits

This is an area where I have seen a few problems. Bulimics who will eat and then vomit often will remove most of the enamel from their teeth because the stomach content is very acidic. It can lead to the need for crowns on all the teeth.

Lemon sucking

Lemon sucking is another way to remove all the enamel. Lemon juice is acid enough that if you like to suck on lemons, you too can be without enamel. Sucking on lemons can become almost an addiction. These patients have a very difficult time stopping.

Soda pop

Letting carbonated beverages sit in your mouth while they defizz can do the same. Carbonated soda is quite acidic and can dissolve enamel. I have heard that if you put an extracted tooth in soda it will remove the enamel. Both diet and regular soda will do the same. Is drinking soda dangerous? Many will tell you it is. I have also read that because when you drink it, it is not in your mouth long so it never has a chance to damage your teeth. There probably are more nutritious things to drink.

> *When I was in the Navy, I had a young Marine sit down in my dental chair. His chief complaint was his teeth were yellow. I looked and sure enough they were. But not because he was not brushing. He had no enamel on the teeth, but only on the*

front of his teeth. I asked about lemon sucking, bulimia, sucking on soft drinks. He answered "No. Sir. I want to look good for inspections so I always brush, but lately it does not help. My teeth stay yellow." I asked, "What do you brush with?", knowing that none of the toothpastes would do this damage but I did not know what else to ask. I had only been a dentist for 3 months.

He said, "Comet."

I said "Comet, like you clean tile with?" suppressing my desire to gasp.

He said, "Yes, it used to get them real white."

I bet it did. It had a component that was an acid, in addition to being having very abrasive particle. He had scrubbed away his teeth. They would never be white again. Now he could have veneers, but at the time in 1964 that was not possible. It must have tasted awful but he wanted to be a sharp Marine and sharp Marines had clean teeth.

Grinding and clenching, popping and clicking, sore jaw muscles or joints

We probably all grind our teeth some at night. Many of us clench when awake and under stress, or simply as a bad habit. This will cause the wearing away of the enamel on the surfaces of teeth that touch other teeth. Let the dentist know if you do this. Actually they will probably guess you do once they look at your teeth.

I have seen farmers who clenched while on their tractors. If you think about this, while on the tractor they were working in their fields often there is a cloud of dust around the tractor. This gets in their mouth. The tractor vibrates and this fine grit, clenching and vibration just simply wear away the teeth. I have seen patients whose teeth are worn down to the gum level. This is almost an impossible problem because you have no tooth left to grip if you crown the teeth. It often requires gum surgery to expose more tooth.

Snap, crackle, pop

Joints that pop and click can cause pain. If it is simply popping and clicking with no pain, you are probably better off not doing anything beyond sleeping in a bite guard. I had one patient who popped so loudly it was embarrassing when he ate in a restaurant. He had no pain and there was no solution.

If you are having pain, that is a bigger issue. The problem is there are many ways to treat this condition, some simple, others very invasive and expensive, and little science to show what is best. Simple is almost always better. Starting with a simple bite guard to sleep in is a good first step.

This and muscle and joint pain falls under the heading of Temporomandibular Joint problems, TMJ, Temporomandibular Dysfunction, TMD, Myofacial Pain Disorder, MPD. There are many experts and every one of them is convinced only their treatment works. Do not under any circumstances let a dentist inject into your jaw joint or stick an arthroscope into the joint, or do surgery on the joint. These are at best last gasp efforts. In general the less you do, the better off you are, but let your dentist know if you are having these problems.

Diabetes

About twice a year the following will happen. I will have a young healthy looking patient sit down in my chair for a filling or extraction. People like late in the day appointments so they can go home after the appointment. This is particularly true if they need a tooth removed.

Half way through the extraction, usually right after part of the tooth breaks, requiring me to do a more involved procedure to remove the tooth, this patient starts sweating, feels cold and clammy. Tells me they feel faint, dizzy, do not feel well.

I check the chart and see a clean medical history. We get a blood pressure and it is normal but their pulse is a little fast. (If you checked my pulse and blood pressure at that point you would find both are high and climbing rapidly. I really hate emergencies.) They are not fainting as the pressure is up so my next guess is low blood sugar. I ask them when they last ate.

"Breakfast, I had a glass of orange juice. I was busy and nervous about the extraction. I skipped lunch."

We cannot print what I say under my breath. I have them drink a can of non-diet soda. I probably join them because my blood sugar is dropping because of the added stress to my already busy day. Within 10 to 15 minutes they are feeling much better and we can complete the extraction. They were having a hypoglycemic, low blood sugar, reaction. It can happen to anyone. It will happen to diabetics if they skip meals. This is almost guaranteed if they take insulin. Insulin is required for them to properly use glucose, sugar. Pair insulin with no food, and they rapidly deplete their blood sugar and we see this reaction.

All too often patients do not feel it is any of my business that they are diabetic, much less what drugs they use to control their diabetes. They did not answer my medical history accurately. This will cause me to be less inclined to think I am looking at a hypoglycemic reaction and they have a much greater chance to go on to a more serious reaction, possibly even unconsciousness.

An even more interesting problem
A young man needed a tooth removed because he had hit it and it split right down the middle. I gave him a small amount of local anesthesia. Sat him upright for it to take effect, talked to him for a minute. He was doing fine, so I went to the next patient while he got numb. Then I heard a scream. Dr. Q! I ran back to the room. The young fellow was twitching all over the chair like he had sat on an electrical wire or had been shot by a tazer. I asked the assistant what happened.

She said, "Just as you stepped out the door he

started doing this, so I yelled and leaned the chair back." That was the right thing to do. I yelled I want the emergency kit now and asked her to get me a blood pressure cuff. By now he had quit twitching and opened his eyes.

"Hi Dr. Q, how are you?" I said I was fine ignoring my blood pressure that was hitting meteoric heights. I said, "You just had a grand mal seizure. Have you ever had one before?"

He, "No, I just dozed off."
I, "No, you had a seizure. " I had checked his chart and again it was clear of any medical problems.

I did not want him driving home until this was all checked out. I was still thinking about sending him to the hospital because he told me this was his first seizure. It was of very short duration, less than a minute, but I was concerned.

I called his wife to tell her I wanted her to come get him and drive him home. He was fine now but should check with his doctor and I would call and explain what had happened.

She said, "Oh, he does that every time he sees blood. He cut his finger last week. I sent him to the bathroom to wash off the blood and told him I would be there in a minute. I heard a thump and went into the bathroom. He had fallen into the bathtub and was twitching like a chicken with his head cut off."

As it turned out it was a faint. The seizure was secondary to the faint, and was probably complicated by the fact that he had not eaten any lunch and had low blood sugar. These reactions can happen to people who are not diagnosed as diabetic or have another undiagnosed problem.

These experiences do add measurably to my production of gray hair. I teach courses on handling medical emergencies in a dental office. My 41 years of experience have given me many examples of what patients did to raise my blood pressure. The Title of the course is, "41 years of Dr. Q's mistakes and how I treated them."

Diabetes and what I need to know

Do you control your diabetes by diet and exercise, oral medication or insulin injection or pump? Do you test your glucose levels on a regular basis? It is very important to let your dentist know that you are diabetic and what you are doing to control your blood sugar levels.

Timing is everything

If you take insulin or sugar lowering drugs, you should ask for early morning appointments right after breakfast, or right after lunch. After a meal, your blood sugar is at its peak and the chance of a low blood sugar episode is low. Do not schedule appointments right before lunch or late in the day. If you must use these appointment times, have a snack an hour before you come to the office.

Let the dentist know the type of hypoglycemic reaction you have, how often, and how to recognize it. The last thing you want is to know your blood sugar is getting dangerously low and not being able to tell anybody because your mouth is wide open and full of dental instruments. Therefore, arrange with your dentist for a signal that will indicate your sugar level troubles. It should be simple, such as raising your hand, and you should remind your dentist each time you are sitting down in the dental chair. Have a glucagon tablet or juice or other treatment handy so they can give it to you immediately.

If you're in trouble, don't wait to let your dentist know. Don't think it will be just a couple of minutes and you can get your sugar taken care of then. The sooner you take care of your blood sugar level, the better for you and for your dentist's stress level.

Asthma

If you have asthma, let the dentist know. Bring your inhaler and show them how you use it and tell them how long it takes to have an effect. As we explained in the section for diabetes, arrange with your dentist for a signal you can use to alert them you need help with your asthma. And use the signal immediately as soon as you detect you might be in trouble.

Rheumatic fever, mitral valve prolapse

Let your dentist know if you have had rheumatic fever, have a heart murmur, mitral valve prolapse, or artificial heart valves. You might wonder why this is important for the dentist to know, but when we clean teeth, do extractions, or some other procedures, we can cause bacteria to enter your blood.

We don't fully understand if this bacteria will cause the problem. But research suggests that if these bacteria lodge on your heart lining or heart valves, they can potentially cause Subacute Bacterial Endocarditis (SBE). SBE can lead to death or the need for an artificial heart valve. While this doesn't happen very often, why take a chance? The remedy is very simple: we pre-medicate you with one dose of antibiotics an hour before your appointment to prevent SBE. However, if you need this pre-medication and forget to arrange for it ahead of time, all is not lost. Simply tell your dentist at the beginning of your appointment. They can administer the antibiotics in the office and wait a while to do the procedure. You'll be okay as long as you get the antibiotics

In April 2007, a paper was published in the **Journal of the American Dental Association** *(JADA) and an announcement was made in the* **American Dental Association** *(ADA) Newsletter from the* **American Heart Association** *that it is no longer necessary to premedicate patients with a few exceptions.*

It will be some time before all dentists and physicians decide just what they are going to recommend. My present plan is to stop premedicating but leave the option open to the patient's physician. If the physician feels they need premedication, the physician should prescribe the medications.

Incidentally, you can cause the bacteria to enter your bloodstream to a lesser extent when your gums bleed when you brush, floss, or bite into hard foods such as apples or cheese. These events do not seem to be a problem and may cause more bacterial exposures each year than your cleanings. Therefore, some researchers question if dentists can really cause SBE. Until research clearly shows we are not the cause of SBE, you simply do not want to run that risk. Be on the safe side and take the antibiotics.

The guidelines for SBE prevention are set by the American Heart Association. Every few years, they review the guidelines and often make changes. There have been at lest five changes since I graduated from dental school and I'm sure there will be more as our knowledge progresses.

Artificial joints

Everything we said in the rheumatic fever section above applies to patients with artificial joints, such as hips and knees. The bacteria can lodge between the bone and your metal prosthesis. If a joint becomes infected, it can take years and thousands of dollars to treat, not to mention the pain you will suffer. The joint can even be lost. To the best of my knowledge this has never happened due to dental treatment but theoretically it is possible. You do not want to risk your new joint. Take the antibiotics. It's a simple precaution.

Heart Problems

If you have heart problems *please* let us know. There was a time when most dental offices were above a drug store. There were no elevators so every patient had to climb the stairs to get to our offices. The trip up the flight of stairs stressed the patient's heart more than most dental procedures. I guess the theory was that if they can get up the stairs, they will be OK.

Today, with modern drugs we are seeing patients with rather sick hearts. Drugs are keeping people alive who simply did not make it in the past. Often we can tell a lot about the severity of your heart problem if you bring a list of drugs you take. If you use nitroglycerine, bring it with you. I'm sure you know this drug gets old after a few months. Therefore it is very difficult for us to keep fresh supplies in our emergency kit. We do our best to keep our supplies current, and we now have a spray that has a long shelf life, but is still makes sense to bring your nitroglycerin just in case.

I frequently see patients who give no history of heart disease, but after I ask they admit they are on 5 or 6 heart medications. They have old, tired hearts, and the drugs keep them going. They often do not realize how little reserve they have. When I look at their list of drugs, I recognize drugs that point to severe problems, alerting me that our appointments must be kept very non-stressful and that I may need to talk to their cardiologists. Not so many years ago many of these patients simply did not live to come to the dentist. Now they live for years and their need for dental care continues but we do need to take special precautions. Bring a list of all the drugs you take for any reason; we really need to know.

High blood pressure, hypertension

A large number of our patients have high blood pressure. This problem is easily controlled with medication. One study of a dental school in Mississippi showed that one third of treated adults with high blood pressure had pressures that were too high. Almost one third of other adults had pressure high enough to need treatment. Sixty percent of adult patients needed their blood pressure to be lower.

We take your blood pressure at least once a year and prior to doing oral surgery. We do not treat high blood pressure. But we want to know if you have high blood pressure because most of what we do will cause your pressure to go up a bit. This could be enough to cause a problem if it is high to begin with.

Just walking into a dental office can raise blood pressure for some people. I suspect that when the mailman delivers mail to a dental office, his pressure rises. Most patients see their dentist more often than they see a physician. We pick up high pressure and refer patients to their physicians on a regular basis, probably at least 2 or 3 times a week. High blood pressure usually does not make you feel bad. Until you have a stroke, have your kidneys quit, go blind, or have a heart attack. I do not want you doing those things in my office. They tend to mess up my day. High blood pressure is easily treated, but you have to get it checked to know if you have a problem.

> *I had a patient come in for a cleaning. He had a pressure of 210/160; we would like to see it below 120/70. I explained I could not clean his teeth; his pressure was dangerously high; he needed to go to a hospital emergency department right then. He was upset. It is just a cleaning, he would check on it next week. I stood my ground and said, No, you are going now. This all happened on Friday. His wife called the office on Monday. My first thought was that he had died or went to some other dentist who said no problem. Instead, she told me they had admitted him to the hospital and his pressure was way down. "You saved his life," she said. "He would not go to the doctor until you refused to treat him."*

Pregnancy

If you are pregnant, your dentist needs to know. Recently there have been many articles in popular magazines and on TV about how periodontal disease might cause preterm deliveries, premature babies. At a symposium I attended, this problem was discussed. Their findings were that periodontal disease, some heart problems, and preterm deliveries were all caused by two aberrant genes. One problem was not the cause of the other. That is, perio disease did not cause heart problems or preterm deliveries. The genes cause a change in our inflammatory system that leads to periodontal disease and the loss of bone around teeth, plaque deposits in our coronary vessels, and preterm labor. Will cleaning your teeth prevent the problem of preterm babies? There simply is no evidence that this is true. It is a genetic problem that leads to preterm deliveries and periodontal problems; one does not cause the other.

Cleaning your teeth will not prevent heart problems

Many dentists have hinted in their Web pages and advertisements that cleaning your teeth can prevent heart attacks and preterm births. As of June 2007 there is no good science to show a cause and effect relationship. When I see the truth stretched by those with elastic ethics, I have a hard time believing anything else they say. Would you really want to go to someone who tries to use scare tactics to con you into making an appointment with them? Do you think they might also exaggerate your other dental needs?

Sometimes the dentist knows first

Some prospective moms will have their gums swell and/or bleed early in their pregnancy. This has to do with their change in hormones and can usually be controlled with very thorough flossing and brushing. There have even been cases where the dentist was the first to know (guess) that a patient was pregnant; however, the EPT tests are more accurate. Generally, it is safer for you and your baby to postpone any unnecessary dental treatment until after you give birth. Note that I said "unnecessary". If you are in pain, you definitely need help.

If you are pregnant and must have a dental procedure, we want to use as little drugs and do as little dentistry as possible. You want good pain control as pain is not good for the baby either. I firmly believe that unless you have an infection or are in pain, dentistry should be avoided until after the baby arrives. Certainly all the elective treatments can safely wait until a better time.

Avoid the first trimester

If you insist on having elective dentistry while pregnant, you should at least avoid the first trimester, the first three months of your pregnancy, as this is when many pregnancies end in miscarriages. It is estimated that as many a 30% of pregnancies end in miscarriages, and often these mothers never realize they were pregnant.

Several years ago a patient came to me for a bridge preparation. I had reserved most of the afternoon to prepare the teeth for her bridge and to prepare temporaries. The patient sat down in the dental chair and said, "I am spending my whole day in doctor's offices." This remark made me sit up. I said, "Really, what is going on?" She responded, "I am 10 weeks pregnant and started spotting yesterday." You can imagine how my hair stood on ends when I heard this. I explained that I did not think we should do anything that day. She went on to her obstetrics appointment, leaving me to read my journals. Sadly, she had a miscarriage that night. This is proof that I am either very good or very lucky to have picked up on her comment. Had I done the bridge as planned, I and probably she would have always believed that the miscarriage was caused by the dental appointment.

We like to avoid the third trimester also because, by then, the baby is getting larger and it is uncomfortable for mom to sit in the chair for a dental appointment. There is always the chance that labor will start in the dental office. We actually had a lecture on delivering children while in dental school. It was described as being much like a quarter back in football, "Just do not drop the ball (baby)." I was never a very good football player so I want to avoid the third trimester. I did "deliver" a baby while in my anesthesia residency, where, while moving the expectant mother from the labor room to the delivery room, she delivered. I had little to do, but it sure increased the speed of the transfer. Again, however, if you are in pain, we must balance the risk of treatment vs. the risk of pain or infection.

I had just such a patient. She was well in to her 9th month of pregnancy. She sat down and it was clear she was expecting. She had a nerve

that was dying and she was having severe
pain. Clearly, she needed help right then and
there. I leaned the chair back and numbed up.
She looked at me and told me she felt terrible.
I looked at her and her skin had all the color of
fresh milk. Her face was cold and sweaty. I asked
for my blood pressure cuff and took her blood
pressure: 80/50, pretty low. Maybe I should take it
again, I thought, I must have made a mistake. The
second measurement was 60/30. My pulse was
now climbing very rapidly. A third measurement
was 50/nothing. I was approaching panic. I had
started her breathing oxygen but this was looking
bad. I looked up and there was her large tummy
sticking up. Duh. The baby was pressing on the
vessels coming from her legs, trapping her blood
in her legs. No wonder she was fainting, not
getting enough blood to her brain. I rolled her on
her side and within 10 seconds her color came
back and she was feeling better. But it took me
a couple of minutes for my pulse to return to
normal. If you know you cannot lie on your back,
tell your dentist.

Epilepsy

If you have a seizure problem, let your dentist
know. Tell them what type of seizure you have
and how often. There are few reactions that
are more frightening to a dentist and their staff,
if they are not expecting it, than a grand mal
seizure. Not to mention it might be dangerous to
you if this happens unexpectedly in the middle
of a delicate procedure.

There are other seizure types that are difficult
to recognize as they amount to nothing more
than a few seconds to a minute of a blank stare.

Warn us so we can take care of you if there is a problem. If you are on medication, let us know. One common anti-seizure medication, dilantin, causes gum overgrowth. Some blood pressure medications also cause a change in gum tissue. If we notice such a change, we might not always connect it to the medication if we don't know you take it.

Osteoporosis

Many of us, as we get older, lose calcium from our bones. This leads to broken bones, hunch back (kyphosis) compression fractures of our vertebrae. There is a group of drugs called Bisphosphonates that are very effective to stop this bone loss. These include Fosamax, Clodranate, Didronel, Boniva, Aredia, Actonel, Skelid and Zometa. Some of these are also used intravenously for some forms of bone cancer. What does this have to do with dentistry? These drugs work by disrupting the healing process of bones. If we extract a tooth or do gum surgery, we can cause large areas of bone to die. This leads to bare bone in the mouth that will not heal. If you are about to start one of these drugs, you first should be sure that all your dentistry is done. This problem continues for years once you start one of these drugs. Their effect lasts for many years. Fortunately, less than 1 person in a hundred on this medication has this happen.

Your family history can also be important

Your health will be the focus of our interest, but

some family history can be important as well. If your parents wore dentures at an early age, it may indicate a history of periodontal disease that has a strong hereditary relationship. (I know, a bad pun.)

Drugs

It's not easy to come out and tell your dentist you are a drug user. Of course it's better to stay away from drugs, but if you use them, it is better to tell. Patients taking cocaine can have severe life-threatening reactions to local anesthesia and to general anesthesia. Methamphetamines are devastating to the teeth. A new syndrome has appeared in recent years known as meth mouth. Those using methamphetamines are seen with large areas of decay in all their teeth. It can completely wipe out a mouth.

> *A dentist I taught with was a professor at a major Western dental school. He would occasionally have prisoners brought to the dental school for treatment. If it was for oral surgery many wanted to be asleep. He would ask them if they had had any drugs in the last 24 hours. To the person they would say "No, I am in jail. I cannot get drugs." He would then explain that if they had any drugs in the last 24 hours and were put to sleep, they would die. Many of his prisoner patients would then admit that even in jail they had managed to get cocaine, some even while in solitary confinement.*

Medications

Bring a list of medications you take. Very few of the medications we use will interact with other drugs except for the sedative drugs we use. Some drugs can be made more potent by other drugs or foods, particularly grapefruit. We need this list to have a second check of what medical problems you may have and to check for drug interactions. By looking at the drugs and reviewing what they are used for we may find a medical problem that you forgot about that could be important to your safety.

A friend of mine had a new patient come in for a cleaning. The patient was in his late 50s. His medical history file showed no medical problems and no record of being on any medicines. The patient sat down in the dental chair and had a heart attack and died in spite of their doing CPR and the fire department's best efforts to resuscitate him. My friend learned later from his patient's family that the patient had suffered a previous heart attack 6 weeks earlier and was on 5 or 6 cardiac drugs. If you will not reveal this information for yourself do it for your dentist. This event really screwed up the dentist's day; he will remember this for the rest of his life, wishing that more could have been done.

Viagra, Levitra and Cialis – Erectile Dysfunction

These three drugs are used for erectile dysfunction, or better sex through chemistry. If you were to have chest pain, we would normally give you nitroglycerine that would cause better blood flow to your heart. If you had used one of these in the last day for Viagra and Levitra, or three days for Cialis, we could not use nitroglycerine as it could cause you to have life threatening low blood pressure.

A patient came to the dentist and needed a tooth extracted but he was petrified of needles. He would not take a shot. The dentist gave him a little blue pill. The patient asked if this would stop the pain. The dentist said no; it is Viagra. It will not stop the pain but it will give you something to hold onto. (the devil made me insert this)

Allergies

Telling your dentist about any allergies you have is very important. It is probably less critical to tell of your pet allergies, but any allergy to medication could change the options your dentist has to treat you.

When you first become allergic to a drug it will usually be an itch or rash. This is bothersome but usually not life threatening. If this happens when you take a medication, you should stop taking the drug and immediately call the person who prescribed if for you. Often Benadryl will be prescribed to control the hives.

It is very important you never be exposed to that drug again or even to similar drugs that may cause a cross-reaction. While the first allergic reaction is usually relatively mild, the second exposure might be the same or it might progress to anaphylactic shock that can be fatal. You dentist needs to know what you are allergic to, particularly if it is to a local anesthetic or antibiotic. Remember, if you ever have to call a dentist after hours, they will not have your chart in front of them, so be sure to tell them again if you have an allergy.

Take control

You life may depend on never being exposed to a drug you are allergic to. Do not trust your dentist of physician to remember your allergies. Whenever you go to a pharmacy to pick up a prescription, ask the pharmacist if this drug is related to any of the medications your have had allergies to. I would feel very bad if you had a reaction and died from a medication I prescribed, but not half as bad as you would. It is your life—take a proactive stance.

Hepatitis and HIV/AIDS

Some of your medical history is used to protect us. Hepatitis can be passed on to us via your blood and saliva. It is also possible that HIV/AIDS could be transmitted that way. We treat all instruments as if everyone is infected. We sterilize all our instruments after each use. We wear gloves, masks, and coats to protect us. However, we will be even a little more careful with the instruments we use with you if we know there is a greater chance of transmission. I do not want one of my staff to get poked while cleaning these instruments. I want to protect my staff as I am sure you do. Don't worry that a dentist will send you away if you tell. If they refuse to treat you because of your condition, they can lose their license.

Let's get reacquainted

Now that we are acquainted, what should you do? Get reacquainted every time we see you. Let us know of any changes in medications, or in medical history or medical status. While I am very good, I am not psychic. If you do not inform me of changes, I will not know. Please keep me current so I can do my best for you.

7. Get to know your mouth

Only God can make a tooth. Any thing I do is, at best, a humble imitation.

We all have teeth and we use them a lot, but we often take them for granted and eventually they start to go away. In this chapter, you will learn about how your mouth works, and what you can do to keep your teeth healthy.

We get 2 sets of teeth

We get 20 primary or baby teeth and 32 permanent teeth if all goes well. The primary teeth are lettered A through T. The lettering starts at the upper right back, across the front to upper left then lower left to lower right. A to J are the upper teeth; K to T are the lower teeth. A, B, I, J are upper molars; K, L, S, T are lower molars; cuspids are C, H, M and R. The rest are incisors.

Do people get a third set of teeth?

There is a portion of the population that have fewer teeth and some amazing individuals who have an extra set of teeth. To the best of my knowledge this is a myth. What probably happened was impacted teeth had been left when the other teeth were removed. Years later these teeth erupted into the mouth giving rise to the idea of a third set of teeth.

Permanent teeth – the ones you want to keep

In the US we number permanent teeth starting at the upper right 1, across to the upper left, 16, then lower left 17, to lower right, 32, as shown in the figure. Permanent teeth have four major classifications, molars, bicuspids cuspids and incisors.

The molars

The molars are in the back of our mouths. They are the grinding teeth and the largest of all our teeth. The upper molars, 1, 2, 3, 14, 15, and 16 will usually have 3 roots that anchor the teeth in the bone. 1 and 16 are wisdom teeth or 3rd molars. Lower molars, numbered 17, 18, 19, 30, 31, and 32, have 2 roots each. They have 4 or 5 cusps on their top surface.

The bicuspids

Ahead of the molars are the bicuspids, premolars. The bicuspids are grinding, tearing, teeth. As their name implies, they have 2 cusps. They will have one or two roots.

The front teeth

The front teeth are incisors and cuspids. The incisors are the front 4 teeth and are used for cutting. The cuspids are the corner, canine/eye teeth, they are tearing teeth. The cuspids have the longest roots of any of our teeth. The cuspids and incisors have single roots.

Let's look at the anatomy of a tooth more closely:

1. The crown is that part of the tooth covered with enamel, that part of the tooth we see in our mouths. Enamel is the hard surface covering the crown. It has a hardness of 80.
2. The root is that part of the tooth in the bone. It is made of dentine. Dentine is the softer material under the enamel that makes up the root and the interior of the crown. It has a hardness of about 20.
3. Pulp is the soft tissue in the middle of the tooth and is composed of blood vessels, nerves and connective tissue .
4. The root of each tooth has a nerve channel, or canal that provides nerves and blood vessels a passageway from the bone at the tip of the root to the pulp chamber in the middle of the tooth.
5. Pulp chamber is the hole that houses the pulp in the middle of the tooth.

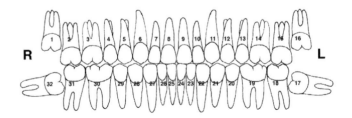

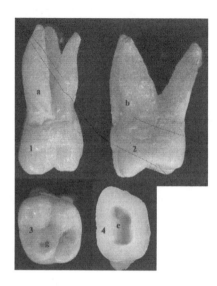

Figure 7.1 The molar tooth

Molar tooth

1. The buccal is the cheek side of the molar. The crown of the tooth 1, 2, 3, that we see in the mouth is comprised of enamel covering dentin. "a". is one of the roots composed of dentin.

2. The side of the molar showing the Buccal, cheek side, roots and Lingual, tongue side root. b, is another root.

3. The top or occlusal surface showing the 4 cusps, points including one cusp that shows wear, g.

4. The inside of the crown cut at about the level of the figures 1 and 2. is the pulp chamber that houses the nerve of the tooth.

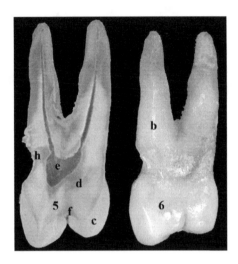

Figure 7.2 The bicuspid tooth

5. shows the inside of the bicuspid, e is the nerve chamber and the nerve canal can be seen leading down the two roots. d. is the dentin that composes the roots and the internal of the crown. c. is the enamel, the hard outer layer of the crown. f is a central grove that did not seal and may have a small amount of decay. h is a groove on the cheek side of the tooth at the level of the gingival tissue. This is referred to as an abfraction and may be the result of clenching.

6 is a side view showing the enamel, crown, and root, b.

The bicuspids come into the mouth around 10 to 12 years of age. They replace the primary molars. A is replaced by 4; B by 5; I by 12; J by 13; K by 20; L by 21; S by 28; and T by 29. If the primary molars are lost early, the permanent molars 3, 14, 19 and 30 can tip forward trapping the bicuspids that have not yet erupted. This leads to crowding of most if not all of the teeth as the child grows.

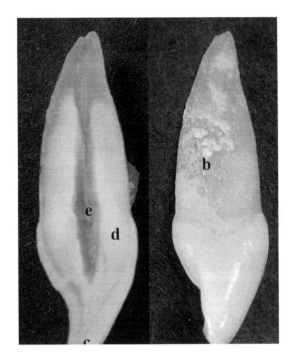

Figure 7.3 The central tooth

c. is the enamel or hard outer surface. b is the root. d. is the dentin making up the root. e. is the pulp chamber leading to the tip of the root.

What happens to teeth

Teeth work hard. They work for a long time. They are important to your appearance, your ability to chew and digest your food and your overall well-being. Dentists spend much of their time restoring teeth. The biggest problem is tooth decay.

Decay

Decay is the loss of tooth structure that results from not cleaning the surfaces of the teeth. It comes in smooth surface and groove decay.

Figure 7.2 5-f. is an example of very early groove decay. Given time these often will go through the enamel layer and spread into the deeper layers of the tooth. The dentine is about 1/4 as hard as enamel so the decay can spread rapidly once it breaks through the enamel. In the case of this bicuspid there is a defect in the enamel but there is still a thin layer of enamel protecting the underlying dentine. There is controversy as to whether such a defect should receive a filling.

5-h. looks like a smooth surface decay that we often see at the level of the gingival tissue in those patients that only brush on major holidays. We also see loss of tooth structure in this area due to the flexion of teeth when patients clench. The decay is soft, the abfractions are hard and smooth. The decay needs to be repaired with a restoration, filling. Abfractions need to be restored once the defect is half way to the pulp. The filling material may be tooth-colored composites, porcelain, silver amalgam, or gold.

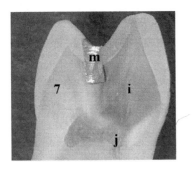

Figure 7.4 This tooth has had decay and received a silver filling, m. The tooth is a bicuspid.

Protecting your teeth

1. If you have teeth keep them. Nothing we do is half as good as what Mother Nature gave you.
2. Clean and floss your teeth regularly. If you will not floss, brush more. If for some reason you cannot brush more or floss, use a fluoride gel every night. This gel can be used even on adult teeth.
3. If you have a dental problem, always ask what will happens if you do not seek treatment.
4. It is your option to have a perfect smile, white, straight teeth. It is also perfectly ok to not go through extensive makeovers.
5. Consider your medical status as a factor in your treatment.

8. Take care of the teeth you wish to keep

One often quoted piece of advice is to only brush and floss those teeth you wish to keep your whole life.

Fluoride made a big difference

Taking good care of your teeth starts before you have teeth. Surprised? Many people are. Yet teeth are forming before a baby is born, even permanent teeth that will not be seen for another 5 years are already forming. So, how do we protect them and make them strong? First, all children should have fluoride in their drinking water. Any municipality that does not care enough to provide this service for it citizens clearly is not interested in its inhabitants' oral health. If you are unlucky enough to live in such a backward city, please add fluoride to your children's juice or milk.

When I was in dental school, all the graduating seniors from Seattle's high schools were examined for decayed, missing, or filled (DMF) teeth. Less than ten percent of all graduating seniors had perfect teeth. Today close to half of each graduating class graduates with no decay, with no DMF teeth. What has caused this dramatic change toward good mouths? Seattle started putting fluoride in its water system in the early 1960s. The children graduating today have had this supplement since they were born. The difference, the year the exams were first done was the same year that fluoride was added to Seattle's water supply. When I started practice, at least half of what I did was fillings, usually 9 to 10 in each new teenage patient and 1 or 2 every year after that. These kids were too old to have the advantage of fluoride in their water while their teeth were developing. Now it is rare to see a teenager who needs any fillings. Less than half will have any decay. My practice has changed very dramatically over 35 years. Therefore, be sure your children are getting supplemental fluoride either in their water or by drops from the time they are born.

Bottled water does not have fluoride. Did you realize that bottled water is more expensive than the gasoline we put in our cars? Often it is no better than ordinary tap water, and in many cases bottled water has been shown to have more bacteria. Tap water is almost free, and if you live in an enlightened city, it will have fluoride. Moreover, consider the cost to the environment to produce, transport, and dispose of plastic bottles. Tap water doesn't cause additional environmental problems.

When do you start brushing?

From the time the child's first tooth arrives, brush it morning and night. We want to get this habit started early. Use a small dab of fluoride toothpaste on the brush. Brush you own teeth at the same time. Children will copy what they see you doing. Let them brush but realize that until they are 10 to 12 years old they will not do an adequate job, so you must help them. Once they have teeth that are close together, start using floss to clean between the teeth. Examine your kids' teeth. If you see white or brown spots, get the child to a dentist.

When should kids go to a dentist?

When should the dentist first see a child? I like to have mom and dad bring them in when they get their teeth cleaned. I want to become friends early before the kids need anything. Usually by the second or third visit the child will let me take a look at their teeth. Often, this will happen before they are a year old. There is a trend to see all kids at their first birthday and regularly thereafter. Most will need nothing, but we do pick up children with early decay. If we start seeing problems by 12 to 18 months, we need to start every possible preventive measure, including fluoride varnish on this child and also on the brothers and sisters and even on mom and dad, because if one family member has problems this early, usually they all will have problems. This is an issue of how often they all brush and floss, what they like to eat, what bacteria they have in their mouths that they share, and genetic considerations, including how strong their enamel is.

When do children need x-rays

By the time they are 3 if we have seen a child

twice a year, we are old buddies. If I see anything starting to develop, I start painting fluoride varnish on the child's teeth. It is faster and more effective than the old way of using fluoride. At about 5 we like to get a complete set of x-rays. We check for decay between teeth, and we look at the formation of roots. We look at the position of permanent teeth. We check for the development of the jaws. This set of x-rays should be repeated every 5 years. We will take posterior bite wings x-rays once a year. We use these x-rays primarily to look for decay between the teeth. We will do it more often if we are seeing decay, less often for clean mouths with no evidence of decay, particularly if the child lives in a city with fluoride in its water.

How often should an adult see a dentist?

In the late 1940's one of toothpaste manufacturers had an advertisement that stated, "Brush your teeth twice a day, have a dentist clean them twice a year." As it turns out, that is pretty good advice. Sometimes I see odd patterns. For example, I have patients who have gum problems or who brush only on major holidays, that I clean every 2 to 4 months. I have others who do such a good job of cleaning, they have no calculus, stain, and never get decay. I can put off their cleaning to 12 to 18 months. I think everyone, even patients with dentures, should be examined at least every 18 months, if for no other reason than to check for oral cancer or precancerous tissue.

Periodontal disease

For those patients with early periodontal, or gum, disease, the most important treatment is getting frequent cleanings. Most gum surgery we all did in the past had little long-term effect that frequent cleanings did not also have. I have many such patients for whom I suggest cleaning every 2 months, and for most periodontal patients I suggest cleaning every 3 months. This will not stop the breakdown seen in severe periodontal disease, but it certainly will help. We will see later that perio disease is probably genetic and made much worse by smoking.

The day I graduated from dental school I knew everything. It was the day I was the smartest I have ever been. I knew everything there was to know about dentistry. We had an instructor who once told us he wanted to apologize that half of what they had taught us was wrong. The problem was they did not know which half it was. We all laughed. We knew better. After 40 years it might have been more than 50% that was wrong. We knew how to cure periodontal disease: you cut off the extra gum tissue, making it easier to clean the exposed teeth and roots. After about 10 years I found these patients again had extra tissue around their teeth but the extra tissue was further down the root because more bone had been lost. The exposed roots we had created were extremely sensitive to hot, cold and many foods.

My quest for the perfect periodontal treatment

I joined a study club that I attended one day a month for 3 years. I read research, I learned the new improved types of surgery, and I did tests. And after all this time I finally knew the answer. Ten year later these people were no better off. They again had periodontal breakdown. Obviously, I just did not have good hands. So I started referring patients to the periodontal specialists. Ten years later they were no better. It is only now that we know that with refractory periodontal disease, those patients who kept getting worse have a genetic disease. Their bodies respond to irritants with an exaggerated inflammatory response. They will start having periodontal problems at a young age, sometimes in their teens, and their bone loss will continue regardless of what we do. The best we can hope for is to slow the breakdown. If they smoke, the breakdown will be even faster. One of the professors emeritus, retired professors, has stated that if periodonts wanted to do treatments that worked they would run smoking cessation programs because that is one thing they can do that makes a real and measurable difference.

X-ray

Even the name, x-ray, is a little intimidating. Why do you need x-rays? How many are too many? How often should you have them? Are they dangerous? What if another dentist took them? What if I don't want x-rays? These are all important and often asked questions.

What if another dentist has taken them?

We will call the dentist and have them send x-rays to us. Provided they are current, we will not need new x-rays or maybe we will need only part of a set to bring you up to date.

Are x-rays dangerous?

We want to keep your x-ray exposure to a minimum. To assure this, we use x-ray machines that have the greatest shielding possible, use the x-ray film that has the shortest exposure time, take as few x-rays as possible, and place a lead apron on you when taking films.

The risk is minimal

A recent paper in the *Academy of General Dentistry Journal* reported on the level of exposure of a woman's uterus when x-rays were taken in a dental office. For an 18 film survey (we take a 10 film survey) the exposure was 0.00001 rad. Your daily exposure due to cosmic rays is 40 times greater, 0.0004 rad. For the panalipse film, exposure is 0.00015 rad, one third of one's daily cosmic ray exposure. You are exposed to 1000 times more radiation from cosmic rays each year than from all your dental x-rays in 5 years. The radiation from one complete set is about the same exposure to radiation form cosmic rays you get flying from Seattle to Miami.

How often should x-rays be taken?

The frequency of x-rays depends on the patient. Patients who are either not brushing well or are having a lot of decay might need x-rays as often as every 6 months. In general, however, I feel the 4 bite-wing x-rays we take of back teeth should be taken every 10 to 14 months. The complete set of 10 films and a panalipse film should be taken every 5 years. Several years ago the American Association of Pediatric Dentists, Academy of General Dentistry, and the American Dental Association set guidelines for how often film should be taken and suggested that bite-wing films should not be taken more often than every 6 months, and full sets of films no more often than every 2 years. We fall well within these guidelines.

What if a patient does not want x-rays?

The guidelines I just mentioned not only set how often we should take x-rays, but also set *standard of care*. *Standard of care* is the level of care that is considered necessary. If I did not take periodic x-rays, I would not be able to know about decay, level of bone, health of bone and roots, the existence of cysts, tumors, impacted teeth. I would not be meeting the established standard of care. In short, I would not be delivering good dentistry. What all this means is I cannot accept or treat a patient who refuses x-rays. If you ever have a question, please ask. But please let me take the x-rays I need to do my job well.

Toothbrushes

In general you want to use a soft toothbrush. It will clean your teeth without damaging your gum tissue. I have seen patients that have scrubbed away much of their natural gum tissue by overzealous use of hard brushes. You can do damage with a hard brush. Change brushes every month, two at the most. Certainly change when the bristles all face in a different direction.

Electronic toothbrushes

These are very important for any patient who has a hard time moving a hand while holding a toothbrush. Do they do a better job? Not if you have normal control of your hands. The Sonicare toothbrush was developed in the Pacific Northwest. It vibrates the brush head at high frequency. The biggest advantage of this brush is the timer. It beeps every 30 seconds for 2 minutes. You brush the upper right side for 30 seconds, then the upper left for 30 seconds, etc. One of the original researchers stated that the Sonicare patients did have more healthy gums than the control using a hand brush. The dentist stated, however, that she felt it was due to the timer. No one brushes for a full two minutes without a timer.

Which is best

There were a number of other similar brushes that came to market. One company would do a study showing they were best. They would then be sued by the other company. Next, another study was done and there would be another round of law suits fighting to determine who was best. While I have no proof, I think they are more similar than they are different. The price range is very dramatic though. I have found battery powered brushes from as low as $1.50 all the way up to over a hundred dollars. There is no convincing evidence that there is much difference.

Proxy brushes

These are small brushes that fit into the interproximal spaces between teeth. These are 1 to 3 mm in diameter, bottle brushes. They do a good job of cleaning under bridges and between teeth that have gaps that food can get stuck in.

Flossing

Flossing is about the only way to clean well between teeth. For children, start flossing their teeth once they have teeth that are close together. You want to start the habit early. The reason is that this is a very difficult habit to start later. My guess is that well less than 1/3 of patients floss. However, many people manage to do a very good job with just a toothbrush.

Three ply baby yarn or superfloss is a good way to clean those large spaces that develop as we get older. The yarn is much less costly than floss. A skein of yarn will last for years. There is also superfloss that is fuzzy like the yarn but is much harder to find. There are plastic threaders that will help you floss under bridges and braces.

Water Piks

About the time I graduated from dental school the Water Pik arrived on the scene. This device sends a pulsing jet of water that you can use to clean between your teeth. It really worked well with inflamed tissue if it was used on low power. It is messy because you are squirting a stream of water into your mouth, and letting the water out the side of your mouth into the sink. It takes a little practice to do it well. If you use a Water Pik, start with body temperature water and use a low setting. You probably never want to use it at higher settings.

Rubber tips

How about the rubber tip on the handle of some brushes? I was taught these were used to exercise the gum tissue. They probably did have some effect, but it was not from exercise. They tended to help clean between the teeth.

Smile Pix

The Smile Pix from Ultradent is a thin plastic toothpick. The sides of the plastic wedge are slightly roughened. These are easy to use with one hand and do a pretty good job of cleaning between teeth. I have found patients and I will use these.

All of these devices work. Some work better than others and your individual needs will be different. Talk to your dentist to see what is best for you.

Remineralization — fluoride

We use fluoride to prevent decay, desensitize teeth, and also to remineralize early decay. One percent neutral sodium fluoride is available over the counter, possibly under the counter. This is a similar concentration that we use for fluoride treatments in the office for kids. One big difference is, in the office we use acidulated fluoride. The acidic pH of this fluoride allows it to penetrate teeth better, and it also makes it taste between awful and just bad. But it works. I do not know of anyone who recommends using it more often than every 3 to six months.

Fluoride gel

The neutral sodium fluoride is about 0.4% fluoride ion. There are other solutions of 1% fluoride, but they require a prescription. The Gel-Kam is a 1% sodium fluoride, making it about 0.4% fluoride. It is available without a prescription. However, because many people mistook it for tooth paste, it is often kept "under the counter" by pharmacists. Ask the pharmacist if they carry this if you do not find in on the shelf.

I suggest fluoride gel for a number of reasons. It works very well to make overly sensitive roots less sensitive. Any tooth that is sensitive to hot, cold, sweet, sour, or salty is a candidate for having fluoride gel brushed on it every day. First brush, floss, rinse and spit as usual. Next, brush 4 or 5 drops of fluoride gel on all the sensitive areas. Swish all around and then spit. Do not eat or drink for the next 3 to 4 hours. The best time to do this is right before you go to sleep.

Remineralizing and preventing decay

Fluoride gels will also harden root surfaces and enamel so there is less chance of getting decay. It probably should be used every day by anyone over 50 to control sensitivity and to assure the exposed root surfaces, which are much softer than enamel, do not decay. As we age, we tend to lose fine motor control of our hands. Many patients over 80 simply cannot do a good job of brushing or flossing. These patients absolutely should use a fluoride gel. Many of us think they should also get fluoride varnish every few months on their teeth and roots.

The magic of fluoride gel

Now for the magic. When a tooth decays, it does not just suddenly have a hole. Decay starts as calcium slowly erodes from the tooth surfaces. As this progresses, eventually enough calcium is lost that we can see in x-rays that the affected area is less dense than other areas of the tooth. Eventually, these areas lose so much calcium they break down and a hole appears. At any time before the hole appears, if you apply fluoride gel on the area every day, you can force calcium back into the tooth structure. In this way, the tooth is returned to better than new. There have been studies that show the remineralized areas are more resistant to decay than the original structure.

Thus if we all brushed with a fluoride gel every night before going to bed, we could probably go our whole lives with little or no decay. We can still get decay in the defects found in grooves in the top of teeth, but that's not a very frequent occurrence.

Be careful with kids

A word of warning: If a child swallows too much fluoride, the fluoride will be added to the forming teeth. As a result, the teeth might erupt with white spots or in the worst case, brown spots. Therefore, keep fluoride gel out of the hands of small children. Generally too much fluoride can leave you with white or brown spots. Fluoride, like many medicines, can be dangerous if too much is swallowed. It can cause fluorosis. Leading to white or brown spots in the enamel. If a small child were to swallow several tubes of Gel-Kam, it could be toxic.

> *Here is the story about how the effect of fluoride was discovered. There were two towns in the Rocky Mountains. The population of one town had beautiful white teeth, but there were several dentists in a town of 5,000 because of the amount of decay people had. The other town 30 miles away was a similar size. The patients had very strong teeth and no one ever got any decay,*

but their teeth were badly stained brown to dark brown. This discoloration problem was blamed on the level of fluoride in the drinking water. This suggested that fluoride might prevent decay, while staining teeth at the same time. Once this was determined, scientists did studies to find the ideal level of fluoride to prevent decay but not cause fluorosis, or discoloration of teeth due to excessive fluoride.

All water supplies should be fluoridated

It is mind-boggling to me that not every town has fluoride in its water supply. It is so simple and inexpensive to add to a water system and has such a major benefit. For some reason anti-fluoride groups fight tooth and nail to keep it out and remove it from cities where it is added. I have heard stories that fluoride is rat poison. It could be at high doses, but it is placed in water systems at about 1 part per million, and at a rate of one drop per 13,000 gallons it is not hazardous to anyone. I have heard it will weaken the bones of the elderly. There is no truth to this. In fact, it has been used to strengthen bones, but at much higher levels. I have heard that if you boil beets in an aluminum pan with fluoridated water and then re-boil them in a copper pan they are poisonous. This is garbage—it simply is not true. I think it was made up by someone who did not like beets.

One school teacher told me fluoridation was a conspiracy of the aluminum companies. She claimed fluoride was a byproduct of the aluminum refining and the manufacturers could not dump it, so they conned the dental industry into advocating that it be placed in our water supplies. This teacher was a flower child of the 70's. She lived on a small farm, grew all her own vegetables, did not drink fluoridated water, nor would she add fluoride to her children's juice. The kids were seeing me because they had decay on most of their teeth. She had pretty good teeth, because she had grown up in a town with fluoride.

Brush your kid's teeth

How can well meaning people keep such a simple treatment from the many children who do not get regular care, whose parents either cannot or will not afford care or supervise their brushing and flossing? I have heard, "A parent should brush their child's teeth." This is true, but many simply do not. I have told parents to brush their children's teeth for three reasons. It will save them money because the kids will not need fillings. This is good for the parent. It will keep the children from having to sit through dentistry. They will have better and stronger teeth. Do it for your child. If you will not do it for you or them, do it for me so I do not have to work on a frightened 3 year old who is going to cry through the whole appointment.

I make it a point to have parents sit in the room while I am treating their children. They need to see just how hard I work. They need to see how kind and caring I and my staff are. They need to sit and suffer with me as their children scream. It is very hard for 3 or 4 year olds to sit through dentistry. Often we have no choice—

the children are infected and need treatment. It is not my fault these children have tooth decay. Mom and dad should suffer right along with me and my staff, and maybe, just maybe, they will get the message.

How can our public officials ignore this major public health problem? It takes courage to be a good public official; obviously many simply do not have the guts to do what is needed. How can people be opposed to fluoride when it does so much good and has no negative effect if it is used properly?

Here are several Web sites that might give you additional information about taking care of your and your family's teeth:

http://www.dentalwatch.org/

Taking care of your teeth
http://www.dentalwatch.org/basic/care.html

Decay prevention
http://www.dentalwatch.org/basic/
mmwr2001.pdf and http://www.dentalwatch.
org/basic/nih.pdf

Fluoride
http://www.dentalwatch.org/fl/fluoride.html
http://www.dentalwatch.org/fl/cdcfacts.html
http://www.cps.ca/english/statements/N/n02-01.htm
http://www.dentalwatch.org/fl/opposition.pdf

9. Kids Kids Kids

Treat a child right and he will be a good patient the rest of his life.

Your first set of teeth

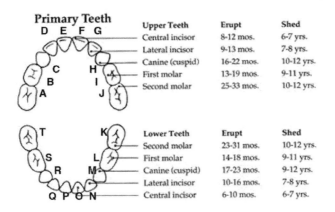

Primary Teeth
D E F G

Upper Teeth	Erupt	Shed
Central incisor	8-12 mos.	6-7 yrs.
Lateral incisor	9-13 mos.	7-8 yrs.
Canine (cuspid)	16-22 mos.	10-12 yrs.
First molar	13-19 mos.	9-11 yrs.
Second molar	25-33 mos.	10-12 yrs.

Lower Teeth	Erupt	Shed
Second molar	23-31 mos.	10-12 yrs.
First molar	14-18 mos.	9-11 yrs.
Canine (cuspid)	17-23 mos.	9-12 yrs.
Lateral incisor	10-16 mos.	7-8 yrs.
Central incisor	6-10 mos.	6-7 yrs.

We get 2 sets of teeth. We get 20 primary or baby teeth and 32 permanent teeth if all goes well.

When will kids get their teeth?

When will your child get his first tooth? Some children are born with teeth. This probably leads to them being introduced to a bottle at an earlier age. Most children see their first teeth at about 6 months. There is a lot of variation in timing. The first teeth to appear are usually the lower front teeth, followed by the upper front teeth and soon after the posterior teeth and finally the cuspids. Small, short, children seem to get teeth a little later.

> *There is an advantage to getting teeth late. We had a neighbor who fell at the age of one and knocked out his two front teeth. So he really never had front teeth until he turned 5. Because he was missing the two front teeth, his permanent front teeth came in early. He fell and broke off the permanent front teeth. He did not lose them but the composite repairs had to be replaced frequently because he continued to break them off. Crowns could not be placed because there would be a good chance of killing the nerve that is quite large at this age. If the nerve died, the root would not properly form and the teeth would be lost. At 22 he was out of contact sports and finally got crowns and had a full smile for the first time in his life.*

> *Perhaps one child in 10 will chip a front tooth. Parents do everything to protect their children and can be devastated when there is an accident. If you have ever watched a one year old walk or a two-year old run, it is the miracle that all kids do not have broken teeth.*

Does diarrhea mean teething?

Children tend to be cranky when teething. Most are pretty miserable for a few days with each new tooth. There really is not much you can do but live through this. Many kids tend to have diarrhea when they are teething. If the child is cranky and has diarrhea, check his mouth.

When they start losing their teeth

Children start losing their primary (baby) teeth at 5 to 7 years of age. Later is better because there is less chance they will break their permanent teeth. The lower front teeth are usually the first to go, followed by the upper front teeth. The molars and cuspids are often still in the mouth at 11 or 12 year of age. Short kids tend to lose their teeth a little later.

Baby teeth have long roots

How is it that baby teeth get loose and are lost (they almost never just fall out)? As a permanent tooth starts to move into its place, the root of the baby tooth is reabsorbed, eaten away by cells in the body. In time when the root is almost completely gone, the tooth will loosen. I remember my parents wondering how teeth with such short roots could stay in place. In fact baby teeth have long roots compared to the size of the tooth we see above the gum tissue. These roots are often quite narrow, making them difficult extractions if they need to be removed.

Kids preserve loose teeth

It amazes me how kids can keep teeth that are so loose they can wave at you. Loose teeth can be hazardous. If a child falls and bumps his head, and if the loose tooth has been knocked out, and then the child inhales, which is the first step to crying, they can inhale the tooth. If this tooth is sucked down into the lungs, it is off to the hospital to recover the tooth. Therefore, for safety reasons, if the tooth is so loose that it will wiggle back and forth 1/32nd of an inch (about 2 mm), get the tooth out.

How I pop out loose teeth

You can remove loose baby teeth at home, but you do so at your own risk. It is better to go to a dentist. Still, if you want to do this, place your fingers behind lower teeth and push down and out fast. If the tooth comes out, it was time. If not, try again in a week. In the past people would tie floss around loose teeth and with a quick jerk it was out. They did not tie the floss to a doorknob. Unless you are accustomed to working in the mouth this is close to impossible to do.

Flip out teeth over a smooth floor, not over carpet or outside. The only thing worse than a loose tooth is losing a tooth. You want to be very sure the child does not inhale or swallow it. In either case you need an x-ray to know where it is. If it is swallowed it will pass on through in a few days, and although the tooth fairy prefers clean teeth, this is not the end of the world. If it is inhaled, it will have to be removed in a hospital. If the tooth is lost in the rug or grass, it can be impossible to find. What are you going to put under your child's pillow for the tooth fairy? But if you do lose the tooth, don't despair. A small piece of white chalk, a chip of white tile, or a very small white stone can serve as a substitute for a small child if you do lose the tooth in the grass. Fortunately for us, the tooth fairy can't see very well.

> *I told one of my patients about this trick with her child in the room. She said the child lost 8 teeth that week, and many of these teeth looked a bit like rocks. She couldn't see any new spaces in the mouth. Some smart kid.*

At one point a dentist was selling plastic forceps for parents to use to "extract" loose teeth. They sold for about $15. I have only seen photos of these. I worry that a parent might try to remove teeth that are not ready. Unless the tooth is very loose, leave it alone.

Why bother with baby teeth?

Is it necessary to take good care of these primary teeth since they will be lost anyway? In a word, yes. These primary teeth hold space for their posterior teeth. If the primary molar teeth are lost early, permanent teeth tend to move forward, locking other permanent teeth from erupting or causing the whole mouth to be crowded.

Around the age of 7 is a time when kids are supposed to look like jack-o-lanterns. However, it is also the time to start orthodontics. The bones are still growing and a little pressure applied can cause additional growth and room. It is much better to get started at this age. Moving teeth is easier, you can gain space, and you get much better long term results. More about this later under orthodontics.

Fluoride, fluoride, and more fluoride

What can be done to protect these primary teeth? First, have fluoride in your water. If your water system does not have fluoride, add it to your child's milk, juice or water. Some vitamins come with added fluoride.

A cup for the first birthday
The most important gift you can give your child on their first birthday is a cup or sippy cup to drink from and the vow to never again give them a bottle!

Baby bottle caries – nursing caries – early childhood caries

Children who are on the bottle or nurse after their first birthday have a good chance of getting **baby bottle decay** which can occur on most if not all baby teeth. The effect of using the baby bottle past age one can be crippling to your child's teeth. It is not uncommon to see a 2 or 3 year old with decay on all their front and back teeth because of their dependency on the bottle. This might be surprising. After all, the liquid in the bottle is the same as the liquid in the cup. But a child can work on a bottle all day, while the drink in the cup will never last that long.

The tragedy is that all the expense and trauma of baby bottle decay can be avoided by simply throwing away all bottles and stop nursing on a child's first birthday. If you will not do it for your child, do it for yourself (not having to sit through treatment with your child) or do it for your child's dentist (they do not enjoy having to restore a mouth ravaged by decay on an uncontrollable child).

There have been several recent reports of decayed teeth that went on to abscess. The abscesses were not treated because the mom could not find a dentist who would take welfare. The infection that started in a tooth spread to the face and eventually to the child's brain. The 10 year old eventually died. All of this could have been prevented with proper home care and a society that believes all children should have dental care. No child should go to bed with a toothache.

Young children are very difficult to treat

To make matters worse, children at a young age have a very difficult time facing dental treatment. Those with baby bottle decay might need work an almost all of their teeth, including fillings, stainless steel or composite crowns, and/or extractions. It is necessary for many of these children to be admitted to a hospital and have their work done under general anesthesia in an operating room. This, of course, can be very costly, hospital charges often being greater than the dental charges.

We are able to treat some of these kids with sedatives in our office. However, this is very difficult, tedious work. Because of their age, even with sedation, these children are not very cooperative. It is not uncommon for the child to move around and cry, even with sedative drugs, making for a very difficult appointment for the child, for the parent, and for the dentist.

Parents do many things to assure their children are healthy, including inoculation against childhood diseases, using car seats and seat belts, ensuring their kids get proper exercise, eat right, and brush their teeth after meals—all important preventive measures practiced by most parents to assure the good health and welfare of their children.

It is our responsibility to do those things that will assure our continued good dental health and that of our children. The best dental care a child can receive is to not need any dental care.

When should children start brushing?

You want to introduce small children to brushing as soon as they get their first teeth. Place a small amount of toothpaste on a soft, small toothbrush and brush their teeth. This is most easily accomplished by sitting down on the side of the tub or toilet. Have the child face away from you standing between your knees. Lean their head back and you have a good view of their whole mouth as it is facing up and if they want to squirm you can hold them between your knees. Brush all sides of each tooth. This is also a good time to floss. Use only a small amount of toothpaste, half the size of a green pea, as they will probably swallow it. Once they get a little older you can get them to spit the extra out. Then let them finish the job. Most kids love to brush. I think they like the taste of the toothpaste. We have to hide the toothpaste from our grandchildren.

The family that brushes together keeps their teeth.

This is also a good time to brush and floss your teeth. If children see you brushing they will want to brush also. It is a good way to get good habits started in your kids and to reinforce your own good habits. Make sure you use fluoride toothpaste.

Now and again we will have a child who starts getting decay at an early age. This may be due to baby bottle, or worse, going to bed with a bottle, poor enamel, bad diet, or genetic causes.

> *How do we examine such small children? We have you hold your child facing you while sitting in a comfortable chair. We sit knee to knee with you. We then have you lean your child back onto your knees. This puts your child's head in our lap with their mouth up. It is now easy to look at their teeth and they feel comfortable because they are in your lap.*

Fluoride varnish and silver fluoride

In recent years we have seen fluoride varnish and silver fluoride come to market. Fluoride varnish is painted on the teeth, particularly the grooves and areas next to the gum tissue. It is orange but this wears off quickly. We are now also seeing a white fluoride varnish that is more acceptable to parents. The varnish holds the fluoride in the grooves that are prone to decay and at the junction of the gum and tooth, which is also a common area for decay. By keeping fluoride in these areas we can prevent decay. We can stop initial decay and remineralize the enamel so the decay goes away. Even if there is a hole in the tooth we can stop the decay in its tracks by placing the fluoride varnish on the area often enough. Fluoride varnish is more effective than the topical fluoride we have used for years. Some parents refuse the treatment because of the orange color that lasts for a few days after the varnish is placed. The new white fluoride varnish is helping with this.

Once we see any decay, we should paint fluoride varnish on the teeth every 2 months. Because decay is caused by bacteria that tends to be shared in families, all the children in the family should be similarly treated, even if they do not yet have decay. If one child has decay, there is a high probability the other kids will also have it as they get older. It is much less costly to prevent decay than it is to repair it. It is also much easier on the child, the parents who have to hold their hands while we work, and yes, it is much easier for the dentist.

Silver varnish in available in many parts of the world. It is painted in cavities and stops them from progressing. It does stain the tooth black permanently, but it is much easier than doing fillings, does not require any numbing, and is quick to place. It has solved major problems in third world countries, where there are few dentists and little disposable income to pay for dentistry. It will be wonderful if and when this comes to the US.

Fillings and stainless steel crowns

What do we do if a child gets decay? Until recently we did small versions of adult fillings. Silver in the back, and composite in the front. If a tooth was badly broken down, we might place a stainless steel crown, cap, over the tooth. These all required that the tooth be numbed. Such numbing can be very difficult for the child, parent, and dentist. It can be almost impossible for a child between 2 and 5 years old. It can be very difficult for some older children also.

ART fillings

Recently a new technique has surfaced known as the Atraumatic Restorative Treatment (ART). In the case where we see a hole in the child's tooth, we scoop out the soft material. We do not go deep enough to remove all the decay or to get to the sensitive area of the tooth. We then seal the hole with one of our newer fluoride releasing materials. This is quick, causes no pain, and leaves the child liking the dentist. The down side is that these fillings might have to be replaced every year or two. However, if we can do this for a 4 year old, and the treatment holds until the child is 6 or 7, many times these primary teeth will be lost before the ART filling needs to be redone.

ART runs against everything I learned 40 years ago. We never left decay; of course we did not have fluoride-releasing material. Treating young children was very traumatic for the kids. Often they had to go to a hospital and be under general anesthesia. This was very expensive. It left many patients with a fear of dentistry.

ART needs to be carefully explained to parents. I tell them I want to remain friends with their children. I do not want them crying, or having pain. I realize these fillings might have to be redone a number of times before the teeth are lost but it is far kinder to the child to do it this way.

Does your child need to see a pediatric dentist?

Is it necessary to go to a pediatric dentist with your children? In one study general dentists who saw children were videotaped treating children, as were specialists who were treating children. These tapes were sent to dentists who did not know the treating dentists who graded the techniques used. Statistically they could not see a difference. They could not determine which dentists on the tape were pediatric specialists.

However, ask the dentist you are considering whether they see children. They will let you know if they would rather not see children. Obviously find someone who treats large numbers of children. It is somewhat more convenient to start as a child with a dentist and continue seeing that dentist through your adult years and even taking your children to the same dentist who saw you as a child.

Special needs children are even more difficult. The skilled practitioner can treat some, but many will need to be seen in a hospital under general anesthesia. I have several Down's syndrome children in my office. We did very well with them. As they get older they tend to have very difficult decay and gum problems.

Sealants

A sealant is a thin layer of plastic that is bonded into the grooves of teeth. When we seal the grooves, food and bacteria cannot cause decay in these very vulnerable areas. A sealant treatment costs about 1/3 to 1/4 as much as a filling. I find that about 1 in 4 or 1 in 5 sealants is lost each year. I really do not like to do things that fail. Are they worthwhile with this great a failure rate?

I was concerned because when my assistants placed sealants, about one in 4 failed by the next year. I took over doing sealants because I knew I was better. One in 4 that I placed failed. I am in a study club with a pediatric dentist. I asked him what I was doing wrong. He said that about 1 in 4 of his fail.

There have been studies where half the mouth got sealant and the other half did not. The researchers followed these patients over years and found they spent less money doing sealants and redoing them than they did doing fillings on the unsealed side. Of course they were also left with more structurally sound teeth on the sealed side. So sealants do make sense.

What we do not know is when to stop treating people with sealants. We seal permanent teeth as they come in. Should we keep replacing these sealants until the patient dies, should we stop at age 18, 22 or 30? I do not think anyone knows. Insurance companies will normally cover them through the teenage years.

Braces – Orthodontics

The American model is that we all have perfectly aligned teeth that are the color of chicklets. Nowhere in the world is this true to the extent it is here. The theory is you will be more successful, more self-confident, more loved if you have a perfect smile. To a certain extent this is true. Some studies show that tall, slim, good looking people with straight teeth make more money. If you are considering a dental makeover, see the makeover chapter in this book.

About 30 years ago, oral surgeons started doing orthognathic surgery to correct mismatched jaw sizes. Where the lower jaw or upper jaw is much larger or smaller than ideal, it may not be possible to move teeth with braces and achieve ideal or even good results. Surgeons can cut the upper or lower or both jaws and reposition the segments to come up with a more pleasing result. In some cases this is the only way to get an ideal result. It may be necessary in some severe cases to even be able to bring the teeth together to adequately chew. This is major surgery but it may be necessary.
See the surgery chapter for more detail.

It is almost socially unacceptable in some communities for children to not have braces. Is it necessary to have straight teeth? Many will say yes, particularly orthodontists. As a teenager, I would have given anything to have straight teeth. But it didn't happen for me and I have done OK. Would I have done better? Maybe. Would I have been a better person? I doubt it.

Tooth prints: Child identification

One of the worst fears we all have when our children or grandchildren are small is that they might get lost, or worse, be abducted. The Seattle Police Department is implementing a program known as Amber Alert. It is activated when a child is reported missing. Reports and photos are immediately flashed to TV, radio, and the message signs on freeways. The goal is to get the message and a description of the child to as many people as fast as possible. There is a place for dentistry to help with this program. We are going to offer tooth prints to all our patients from 3 to 18 years old or to any patient who feels they need one.

What is a tooth print?

We place a putty-like impression material on your child's teeth and have him bite down. This impression sets to a rubbery consistency in about a minute. The material we use does not change shape after it sets. The shape and size of teeth do not change. The impression is a permanent record of the shape of your child's teeth. This impression can be used as proof of the identity of a child. Teeth and their arrangement are every bit as individual as our fingerprints. Children will lose their baby teeth. For this reason, we think we should take an impression at age 3 to 6, again from 6 to 10 and a third impression after children have their adult teeth.

There is another major advantage to the impression. Our saliva is a great source of our scent. If a child gets lost, you can take the impression and it will give tracking dogs a good scent to use when trying to track down a missing child. The scent doesn't last forever, but it does last a long time.

How does this work

We take the impression. We have you write the name of your child on a zip lock bag. We place the impression in the zip lock bag, and you take it home and place it in a safe place. We encourage you to also place a recent photo of your child in the bag, one that shows your child's face and the clothes he normally wears to school. If you ever need a photo, you want one you can get to quickly.

A DNA sample

We will also rub your child's cheek with two Q-tips. These will be put in a separate zip lock bag. This bag should be placed in your freezer. This will serve as a sample of DNA that can also be used to identify a person. Do not put the bag with the impression in the freezer, just the one with the swabs. Frozen saliva does not work as well for tracking dogs.

We can take the impression at your child's next fluoride appointment. If you want it done before your recall appointment, call and make an appointment. All of the ideas may not be appropriate for the very young children; talk to your children about the ideas that you feel are appropriate.

What does it cost?

This community has been very good to me. I feel this is a very important program. This just takes a few minutes and a couple of dollars for materials. We want all of our young patients to have this protection; so, we are not charging our patients for performing the impressions or the swabs. The cost is mostly materials, and it should be under $50 if you request such a service.

Hopefully no one will need to use any of this. I will be perfectly happy if I waste the material and bags. However, if it ever makes a difference, I would be very thankful I took the precaution.

It is too late to collect the information if we wait until it is needed. Do it now.

While we are talking about things that no one wants to talk about let's look at a further child safety issue. While this is not strictly dental it is so important we thought it should be added to this chapter.

Safety suggestions for your children

Your children should know their full name, address, and telephone number including area code. The parent's work numbers is also helpful and good to know. Make sure they know how to call the operator and make a long distance call.

Tell your children to always stay with a friend or group of people and never go to isolated places.

Children should never be left alone in a car or in a supermarket cart.

Explain that grownups do not need to ask children for help. If a stranger asks them for help, it is best to ignore them, leave the scene immediately, and tell a parent about it.

Teach children they must never accept candy or presents from someone they don't know.

Children's names should not appear on clothing or other personal articles where a stranger can easily see it. A child is more likely to respond if called by name.

Tell your child to go to a checkout counter or clerk when separated from you while shopping—never the parking lot.

Instruct day care providers, baby-sitters, or other caregivers not to release your child to anyone but you without your permission.

When home alone, a child should not answer the door or tell someone over the phone he or she is alone.

Have your child agree to call you should he or she change agreed upon plans.

Know your child's route to school, friend's houses, and friends.

Observe what your child is wearing every day.

Teach children they can and should say no if an adult makes them uncomfortable, or if an adult asks them to do a something wrong, touches them inappropriately, and so on.

What to do if someone tries to abduct your child

Tell your child to kick, scream, and fight if a stranger tries to force him or her to do something. They should yell, "This is not my daddy or mommy."

If they are abducted, tell them to leave hair in the car and smear saliva over the door handles and other places in the car.

What if they get lost in the woods?

Keep spitting

If they are ever lost, such as in the woods, tell them to spit. There is nothing a child wants to hear more than it is OK to spit. If kids will keep spitting, search dogs can often smell saliva.

Hug a tree

Next, teach them that if they are lost, they should sit down and hug a tree. Search crews will find children if they will stay in one place. If they keep moving it can be very difficult.

What can you do to help?

- Look at your child's teeth. If you see white spots, these are early decay and we need to start applying fluoride varnish immediately. If you see holes we need to place ART fillings. Do not put off treatment, it will only get worse.
- You need to stop nursing the child at age one. The child also needs to stop using the bottle at age one. Both of these will lead to early childhood caries ECC or nursing caries.
- Every morning and every night place a small amount of fluoride toothpaste on a brush and brush your children's teeth. They may want to brush and it is OK to let them, but they will not get their teeth clean by themselves. It is important to do this as soon as you see teeth. If you cannot brush, put a small amount of fluoride toothpaste on your child's finger and rub it over the teeth.
- If any of your children have had decay, brushing becomes even more important for the brothers and sisters, because they will have decay sooner or later.
- Try to give your children snacks that contain low sugar and try to limit them to two or three times a day.
- Take your children to visit a dentist when your children are about age one. Ask your dentist if he minds you bringing your children to your cleaning appointments.

Better to get to know the dentist early.
- Talk to your child about what they should do if they are abducted.

HERMAN®

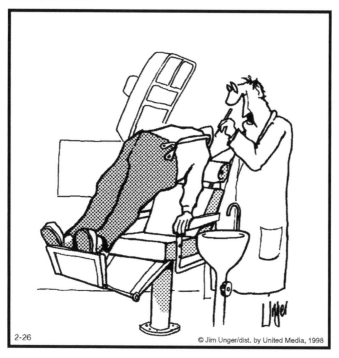

2-26

© Jim Unger/dist. by United Media, 1998

"Try to relax."

10. Pain in the night: Dental emergencies

My threshold for pain is much lower than my dentist's

What is a dental emergency?

It is a condition that if left untreated will lead to further breakdown, a worsening of the dental disease, is giving you pain that cannot be controlled with aspirin or ibuprofen, or could lead to death. My threshold to declare an emergency in my mouth may be less than the dentist. *It isn't, see more later*.

Some things need immediate attention. If you have a tooth knocked out you need to be seen immediately. If you have been in pain for a couple of days and cannot get to sleep, you probably can wait until tomorrow. It really is not fair to call your dentist at midnight if you have been in pain for two days and could have come in during office hours. If you are running a temperature say over 100 degrees F, you should at least talk to your dentist and get on antibiotics. If you are swelling, particularly if it is swelling below the edge of your lower jaw, floor of your mouth, or if you eye is starting to swell closed, you need to be seen now.

Do I take my own advice?
I am on our disciplinary body. I was on a case 60 miles from my home and my dentists. On the first day I had a tooth develop extreme pain. I got

some Aleve and took more than I should have but got the pain under control. If I had left to go to a dentist, the hearing would have been put on hold. The judge, attorneys, and expert witnesses would have had to wait. The case could have been dismissed. I got to sleep the first night at about midnight and was up at 5 for more Aleve. The second day, I went to a pharmacy and got some ibuprofen, which is very good for tooth pain. That held me through the next two days. Clearly I had a tooth dying and needed a root canal. I thought about prescribing some antibiotics for myself but that is quite illegal; I could end up before the board. On the 4the day, we finished the case and I stretched the speed limit a little to get to my dentist. He opened into the pulp chamber and said, "that is a lot of puss, Fred, you should have been able to walk on water with all the pain."

Well not quite but I was getting close. I was a bit stupid and quite lucky. I could have ended up with a very serious infection.

Knocked out or displaced tooth

Should you ever have a tooth knocked out or moved out of position you have a true dental emergency. This is one case where it is important to get to a dentist fast. If the tooth is still in the socket but is displaced leave it in the socket. These teeth can be repositioned rather easily if you are seen within an hour or so.

If the tooth is knocked completely out of the socket time is very important. The sooner the tooth is put back in place the better. Before you leave for the office, the tooth should be rinsed in tap water. *Do not scrub or wipe the root.* It should not be touched. Leave any tissue attached to the root where it is. Look at the root to see if it is broken or cracked. Do not worry if the crown is cracked. If everything looks OK put the tooth back in the socket. Bite your back teeth together and hold the tooth in place with your fingers. If you cannot bring yourself to place the tooth in the socket or if it has a cracked or broken root put it in a glass of ice water that has a pinch of salt and *get to a dentist quickly.*

Of course, if the tooth is a baby tooth it may just be the normal process of being lost so that it can be replaced by a permanent tooth. Your best guide is if the tooth has a root that is more than a quarter of an inch long you should be seen immediately.

I had a patient call me one Sunday morning because she had dropped her denture and broken one of the front teeth. While this was an emergency for her, It really was not life threatening. All I could have done was try to Superglue it in place. No dental lab is open on Sunday. I told her what to do and she was able to Superglue it in place. She came in on Monday and we sent it to the lab for a more permanent fix. Superglue will sometimes work on dentures. You fix the denture on a sheet of paper, not in your mouth. This fix is temporary, however. Follow all the safety suggestion that come with super glue.

Dental pain

If you are having pain it is usually and indication that something is wrong. It may be a tooth, the gingiva (gums), the bone, the jaw joint, or the muscles that move your jaw. The first thing concerning most patients is relief. Aspirin, Tylenol, or Advil are good pain relievers and should be tried first, provided you can use them. *They only work by swallowing them. Never put either on the tooth or area that is bothering. They will burn the lining of your mouth.* If these fail, the next thing to try is ice water. This will often stop the pain of a dying tooth.

Swelling

Should any part of your mouth, lips, or face start swelling due to a dental problem you should also seek help as this often is caused by infection. If the swelling gets bad enough that your eye starts to swell closed, you start having trouble swallowing, or you start running a temperature, you need to be seen immediately.

Getting help

Your dentist is required in most states to have coverage 24/7. A note on the answering machine to call the local hospital is not adequate. Physicians are very smart but most do not know much about teeth.

My office always used the following

You should get help for all of these problems. During office hours call the office. At night or on weekends you can call our emergency pager and when asked, enter your phone number. Hang up. This will trigger the pager and one of us will call you back. This number is also on the office answering machine so you can get it by calling the office. It is also listed in the white pages of the phone book.

It did not always work
I had a patient come in one Monday morning in pain. He said, "you doctors and your unlisted numbers." I told him my name was in the phone book. He said, "It is not. I looked two times on Saturday." I went and got the phone book and showed him. He had looked in the phone book and had given up when they got to the Quanstroms thinking that the rat had an unlisted number. I am listed, but the Quarnstroms a little further down the page in the listings. You must spell rat with an R.

I later added the spelling Cornstrom and Kornstrom. I wanted patients to be able to contact me.

Should you not be able to reach me, the University of Washington Hospital has a dentist on call that can see you. (We have had the pager fail a couple of times.) Hopefully, you will never need any of this information.

Should your dentist's answering machine say to call the local hospital, I would consider finding another dentist.

11. Scared – don't be.
The fear of dentistry

There are two kinds of dental patients. Those who admit they are frightened and those who will not admit they are frightened.

There is very little we do as dentists that does not involve some pain. We learn as small children to avoid things that cause pain. There are a few who enjoy pain and you will find them in counseling or institutions.

The common level of fear varies from, I really do not like to go to absolute paralyzing levels of fear. There have been studies that show roughly a third of the population avoids going for dental treatment because of their fear. Studies have been done in different ethnic groups and this finding is universal in many cultures.

How can this be? Dentistry in the last 40 or 50 years has made giant strides in fear and pain control. Local anesthesia is much better than it ever was in the past. We have oral medication that helps with apprehension; it is even possible to have intravenous sedation or general anesthesia. Yet, patients are still fearful.

Find a dentist who cares

Rule one for the apprehensive patient. Find a dentist who is not afraid of you, someone who not only cares but also has some special skills to help you be relaxed. Many of my colleagues simply do not have the skills or temperament to work with fearful patients. This is not surprising if you look at dental school. We spend 99% of our time learning physiology, anatomy, biochemistry, periodontics, endodontics, surgery, and restorative dentistry. If we went to a very progressive school we got to spend a week in a fear clinic seeing phobic patients treated by the experts. Certainly we would never take on someone like that. I was having trouble enough trying to learn to do fillings, crowns, and root canals, much less do them on a moving, crying target.

I had dinner with one of my classmates. We got into a discussion of fearful patients. He said, "Fred, you can treat anyone if you just take the time to talk." I retorted, "I have patients who will not even come and see you if they know you do not do at least nitrous oxide to help them relax."

"That is silly, I can treat anyone."

As dinner progressed our "discussion" got louder. Our wives rolled their eyes and said we really should not let these two get together, much less after a drink. Another glass of wine and the wager was made. I had a patient who needed, but could not afford, a crown. I would refer her to him. If he completed the crown, he would win and I would pay for the crown. If he could not complete the crown I would complete it, giving the patient sedation and he would pay for the crown. The loser would also pick up the tab for our next dinner.

I called the patient and explained that the dentist was very kind, very caring, and very gentle. And she could get her crown at no cost to her. After she stopped laughing and told me I was out of my mind if I thought she would let any dentist touch her mouth without some sedation, she politely told me no thank you. She would save up and have the crown done with sedation.

The psychology approach

So what can be done? There are fear centers in many dental schools. Psychologists work with patients to desensitize them to the dental techniques, tools, and equipment. First is getting them to the clinic, next is sitting in the dental chair and just looking around. The patient is always in control. The patient can refuse or delay treatment at each step. The next step is to have the patient handle the instruments that will be used. They are even encouraged to hold the anesthetic syringe. They practice having an injection with no needle. This may take many appointments but, eventually, many are able to cope with techniques that are taught and are able to sit for dentistry. This does require a very patient dentist who is willing to go very slowly and who is trained in using these techniques.

All types of people have fear

It should be emphasized that this level of fear transcends all cultural, economic, and racial categories. From the welfare patient to the industry CEO, from the high school drop out to the college professor. You will find patients who have not been to a dentist for 20 years. Some patients are simply too fearful or will not take the time for this technique to work. It often will involve 5 or more appointments with the psychologist before any work is done.

Most dental students graduate not realizing just how common dental fear is or how devastating it can be. Our patients while in school were screened to be easy to work with. We were learning it was tough enough to do simple filling much less spend 4 hours with psychological relaxation techniques that we did not know. We graduated ready to wipeout decay and dental disease and soon discovered that no one cared. The most dreaded phrase in the English language is, "This is your dental office. It is time for your appointment."

My first exposure to dentistry was as a Navy dentist serving the Marine Corps. I doubt if I will ever forget the phobic Marine who sat in my dental chair my first week in practice. He was over 6'4" his arms were bigger than my thighs and their size was due to muscle and not flab. He sat in the chair; rather, he suspended himself in the chair with only the back of his head and his heels touching the chair. His body was rigid. In addition, he was the company-boxing champ. This was a patient I did not want to hurt. We talked the first appointment. He described some terrifying appointment he had as a child down South.

We talked the next appointment. Not that I was so skilled a talker, I was afraid to treat him. I now knew the fear of dentistry, not as a patient but as a provider. He could break me in half. I eventually got my courage up and we cleaned his teeth. I was very relieved he did not need any fillings.

The Navy next sent me to Vietnam to make the first amphibious assault across a beach by American forces and to treat patients with a drill powered by a foot treadle, much like old-fashioned sewing machines. Here I was my first year out of school with few of the tools I considered necessary to do dentistry.

I also did some people to people dentistry on Vietnamese. We would pick a squad of marines and hike 3 to 5 miles through rice paddies to small villages. Probably the most dangerous thing I have ever done. We would go to small villages and do extractions. There were no dentists for 200 or 300 miles. Dental infections were common, many with severe swelling, and in some cases life threatening.

My first trip to the village was eye opening. Almost immediately we had 20 potential patients lined up. I went down the line examining them as best I could. I had no x-rays, no medical history, and only the dental instruments I could carry. I spoke no Vietnamese. They spoke little or no English. They would point; I would look and we would try to communicate by pointing and mimicking what I would do. I numbed up the first 10 and started to work. One of the teachers came and asked what I was doing. I explained I had put their teeth to sleep so I could remove them without pain. He responded to not do that. They thought they would be that way the rest of their lives. They were all about to leave. I explained they would return to normal in a couple of hours. He told me not to do that. The pain did not bother them. I just pulled the offending teeth on the next ten patients. They did not grimace, tense, or make a sound. I was in a cold sweat. The teeth were all badly infected so they came out easily. We could work for about 2 hours and then had to get out of the village because that gave the Vietcong time to react to our presence. In fact, probably many of my patients were VC. I saved lives every time we went to the village because many of the patients had very serious infections. However, if I had treated patients like that in the US I would have been sued. No anesthesia, no x-rays, no medical history. Wipe the forceps off with alcohol between patients. Yet I am probably more proud of my trips to the villages than any other aspect of dentistry I have done. I literally saved lives every day while there.

Everyone perceives pain differently

This illustration points out that different people perceive pain differently. After my 2 years in the Navy I was a civilian and still a bachelor not ready to settle down so I took the first year of a Medical Doctors Anesthesiology residency. I spent a year in a hospital in Washington DC giving and learning general anesthesia. I put somewhat over 1000 patients to sleep for surgery. When I was on call I also gave anesthesia for deliveries, one of my greatest thrills. It is so exciting to see a life start. I also went to all the cardiac arrests that occurred in the hospital at night when I was on call. It was a large hospital, with a lot of old and very sick patients. It was rare to not attend a cardiac arrest each night on call. It was a good year and I learned a lot.

Is general anesthesia hazardous

It had been my goal to be able to put fearful patients to sleep, under general anesthesia and do their dentistry. Go to sleep and wake up with all the dentistry done, what a dream. My residency was a little too thorough. While I never lost a patient, it was made clear to me that there were some risks to general anesthesia. As my department head stated, in anesthesia we may only lose one patient in 700,000 anesthetics, but it is 100% for that patient. I finished my residency and set up a practice to treat fearful patients.

The turf wars

What a rude awakening. I thought I might like to teach a day a week at the dental school. My year's residency was quite rare and I expected I would be welcomed with open arms. The head of the oral surgery department sat me down and picked my brain. I had used IV Valium that was just coming to market and looked to be much safer than the commonly used pentethol. I had been fortunate enough to have used it in a study that led to its FDA approval. After discussing all the variety of cases and drugs I had used, he said, "Do not ever get into trouble doing anesthesia, as I will probably serve with the prosecution." I asked, "Why would you say that? I had 4 times the training your oral surgery residents get. In fact, I helped supervise them." He said, "Yes but anesthesia is not a dental specialty. You are not a specialist. My surgery residents will be specialists in oral surgery."

Welcome to the world of turf wars. The surgeons were and still are paranoid that if general dentists can sedate patients, they will also do extractions. Surgeons consider this to be their turf. About this time, hospitals started requiring that a physician do the history and physical on all patients that were admitted to a hospital for surgery. This meant that the Oral Surgeon had to have a physician admit the patients they took to the hospital. Within a few years, Oral Surgery residency programs started granting an MD degree to all their residents. They have similar training but do not take the full medical school that would lead to an MD. I have had many friends and patients say, "My oral surgeon is also a "Dr." referring to their MD." They have an MD but they did not complete medical school. Many of the older surgeons are simply DDS or DMD, dentists. In many cases they are better surgeons than the DDS/DMD MD surgeons. There is no difference in their training.

The path to the specialty of Surgery is a long one. It can take as many as 4 years after dental school, possibly more if research is done. I know of surgeons who will charge for up to 3 hours of anesthesia each hour. They are charging for general anesthesia when they are not with a patient. Not only is this illegal, it is dangerous. The surgeon should be with the patient full time from the time they are put to sleep until they are awake. You should not be left with a nurse unless they are a certified nurse anesthetist. You should never be left with a dental assistant while you are under general anesthesia.

DMD vs. DDS

While we are on the topic of degrees, what is the difference between a DDS and a DMD, Doctor of Dental Surgery vs. Doctor of Medical Dentistry? The answer—no difference. Some schools give one degree; other schools give the other degree, but the training is the same.

Local anesthesia

Let's look at the wonderful area of anesthesia, painandfearcontrol.Itissomewhatcontroversial as to who was the first to do anesthesia. Dentists believe it was Horace Wells using nitrous oxide. Physicians believe it was a physician in Georgia who used ether for general anesthesia. As the story goes, Wells saw Colton, an itinerant lecturer, administer nitrous oxide at a lecture. The person receiving the nitrous oxide barked a shin and was injured but had no pain. At this time dental and medical surgery was done with no anesthesia. You hoped your dentist was fast because there was nothing for pain. Some of the more advanced would administer alcohol or laudanum, a narcotic mixture.

A dentist does general anesthesia

Wells was impressed. He used nitrous oxide as a general anesthetic for the first time in 1844. He started doing extractions using just nitrous oxide. It was years later that it was discovered it was important to also administer oxygen. However, these early dentists were very fast so the patients were not asleep for very long. It was a major advancement for both dentistry and medicine. It was even more remarkable in that witches were being dunked in Salem, Massachusetts only a few years earlier. It was a quantum leap for mankind to stop killing witches and to turn our efforts to pain control in Boston only a few miles and a few years later. Local anesthesia came along in 1884. A physician used cocaine to numb the eyetooth, cuspid. Modern local anesthetics have no chemical similarity to cocaine, although cocaine is still used for some very specific types of topical anesthesia.

Every dental office should offer empathy and caring to their patients. With a proper atmosphere, many fearful patients can be treated with local anesthesia and a kind word. The fact that a dentist shows concern will go a long way to help those who are slightly nervous.

It is important to let your dentist know you are apprehensive. I had a hernia repaired a few years ago. Because of my anesthesia knowledge, I am very uptight about anesthesia. I told the anesthesiologist and she quickly gave me something to relax. It is OK to let us know. We do not give medals for bravery. If you do not tell us, we may not know.

HERMAN®

by Jim Unger

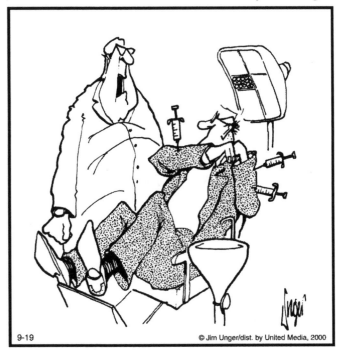

9-19 © Jim Unger/dist. by United Media, 2000

"WILL YOU PLEASE KEEP YOUR ARMS DOWN!"

We don't use novacaine

Local anesthesia has done a lot to help with patients' fears. It is very very rare to have a case where local anesthesia does not give complete pain control. First, our local anesthetics are very good. These are commonly known as Novocaine. However, we have not used Novacaine, procaine, in dentistry for years. It is an ester, and patients are prone to allergies with its use. It has a number of side effects we do not want to face like methehemoglobinemia. But most important, it is not a very profound anesthetic. It does have some valid uses in medicine when used for spinal anesthesia.

Xylocaine

Our most common local anesthetic is xylocaine, lidocaine. This is probably our safest local anesthetic. It comes with several dilutions of epinephrine. The epinephrine gives it a longer effect. The epinephrine causes small blood vessels to constrict slowing the reabsorption of the xylocaine. This gives us a couple of hours of profound anesthesia. However, the epinephrine can also make your heart beat a little faster and give you a shaky sensation that lasts a few minutes, if we get it close to a blood vessel. We have to be close to the nerve or we will not get anesthesia; unfortunately, often blood vessels run with the nerve. This anesthetic is the least toxic of all anesthetics. We can use up to 10 cartridges in an adult patient. I cannot imagine the necessity of using this much in one appointment. I would look for a dentist with a little better aim and knowledge of anatomy if they are using this much.

Xylocaine is by far the safest for children. It follows the rule of 20. For every 20 pounds a child weighs you can use one cartridge. If your dentist is numbing up your child's whole mouth they will use 4 cartridges. That is a bad idea for several reasons. First, children must weight 80 pounds to be able to tolerate this much. Second, if you numb the whole child's mouth, your child will probably chew up his lip and cheek and tongue because it feels strange and it does not hurt when they bite it. One side or even just one quadrant upper right, upper left, lower right, or lower left is enough at one time. The children become good patients if you go slowly. Several shorter appointments are better than one long one. Each time a child has a good appointment, the next one becomes easier. There have been a number of deaths of children who were given sedation and then the dentist numbed up the whole mouth. At first, these were blamed on the sedation. It now appears that it had more to do with the amount of local anesthesia given than it did the sedation. However, when we talk about Chloral Hydrate, you will see it may have been a combination.

I could spend another 5 pages writing about the various anesthetics. Suffice it to say, we have one that will keep you numb for 6 to 10 hours. Why would you want to be numb for 10 hours? If you have an extraction and Marcaine, bupivacaine, is used, you may not need any other form of pain control. Most pain from dentistry is the result of swelling. Most swelling happens within the first 6 hours. If we can keep you numb for the first six hours, Tylenol or Advil is probably all you will need for pain control.

Septocaine, articaine

In the last 10 years, we have a new kid on the block. Septocaine, articaine, came on the American market after being available in Germany for about 20 years. They have done a masterful job of marketing. Dentists think it is magic. Almost all of dentistry thinks it is better than the other anesthetics. Several researchers have attempted to show it is superior. No one as of this writing has managed to show any advantage. You can believe that the manufacturer will send us a copy of the paper if one is ever published. There is one researcher who may have managed to show in the pure research setting that it is a little better.

He took the favorite dental research animal, dental students, and injected them with two different anesthetics in the lower front of the mouth. The injections and solutions were random and not known to the dentist giving the injections. He did show a slightly better effect with Septocaine.

So why not use it? It comes in a 4% solution. There is one other 4% solution, Citanest, prilocaine. Citanest is another one that can cause methehemaglobin anemia. However, both 4% solutions are known to cause paresthesia, your lip remains asleep for a long time, if not the rest of your life. The incidence of this is very low, about 1 in 200,000 blocks but that is 20 times greater than xylocaine. But it is 100% if it is you.

You may drool the rest of your life and kissing will not be much fun. Pucker up. Of course I will not be able to enjoy the kiss because my dentist used a 4% solution. Unless you have a unique problem it might be better to use the safe anesthetic, xylocaine.

How about electronic anesthesia?

A few years ago, several companies came out with the solution to local anesthesia problems. You hooked up a couple of electrodes either in the mouth or on the skin of the cheek. The patient was given a control and encouraged to increase the electric signal to as high a level as was comfortable. These machines were powered by batteries and were a not too distant cousin to the TENS machines used in medicine for sore backs, necks, and other aches and pains. In fact some of the machines were TENS machines. It looked good for a while. In fact, I was able to do a lot of fillings and even some crowns with these machines. However, the failure rate was about 40%, way too high to be practical. If you added some nitrous oxide, laughing gas, the success rate climbed to about 90%. Close but no cigar; a 10% failure rate is not acceptable.

One of the things I learned after failing with the TENS machine was that patients felt much less pain when getting the injection to be numb after I had failed with the TENS machine. There was some research that showed the electronic signal was much better than topical anesthesia for blocking the pain of the injection.

Topical – the stuff they paint on your gums

How about topical anesthesia? The tissues feel numb to a finger after painting the topical anesthesia on tissues. However, this anesthesia is only very superficial. You cannot get the bevel of the needle through the tissue without it being felt. There is one exception, EMLA. EMLA, a eutectic mix of local anesthesia, is a mix of xylocaine and prilocaine. It has been shown to penetrate skin, something that other local anesthetics will not do. It is better for the tissues of the mouth also. With the exception of EMLA, I know of no topical that has shown to be better than flavored Vaseline in true double blind placebo controlled studies (real research). Placebo is a very big factor in pain control. If you rub bat guano on patients' noses and tell them their lips will be numb, something like 30% of people will report numbness. Not that I ever did this.

The wand

Enough for the stuff we rub on gums. What else can be done to make injections better? One company sold a device that was computer controlled. It made the injections go verrrrry slooooowly. The slower you go the less you stretch the tissue and the less pain you have. The problem was that this machine was so slow, I could take a nap waiting for it to finish. I did not feel it was better than just injecting slowly and it cost almost $2000.

The vibraject

Another company came out with a vibrator that fit on the syringe. This did help get the needle through the tissue and helped make the injection less painful. It was less costly, about $350. No wonder dentistry costs so much; $350 for a vibrator about the size of your little finger. What else can we do to make the injection less painful?

Let the dentist know

It is very important to get good numbness with all patients, particularly children. Should you ever have pain, let the dentist know. Now and again we will have a patient that, despite our best efforts, still has pain. These patients need sedation along with local anesthesia.

Nitrous oxide sedation

The most common sedative in dental offices is nitrous oxide. This is the same gas Dr. Wells used to give the first general anesthetic. It turns out to be a very poor general anesthetic but a great sedative. It is breathed through a small nose mask. Patients will have the sensation of an alcoholic beverage or two but the effect wears off very quickly, so there is no problem with driving home after an appointment. We typically use mixes of 30 to 40% nitrous oxide and 60 to 70% oxygen.

It gives good pain control, and in moderated amounts of sedation, the patient is given 3 to 4 times the amount of oxygen found in room air. This gas has also been used to transport heart attack patients in the ambulance. It is very safe. There are only a few patients who cannot use it. These include those with advanced lung disease, known as Chronic Obstructive Pulmonary Disease, COPD. We would prefer not to use any sedatives with those who are pregnant.

Hallucinations

Once in a great while we will have someone hallucinate while on nitrous oxide. This can be frightening for the patient and the dentists. The solution is to take the mask off and go back to breathing room air. They quickly return to normal. Very rarely women have sexual hallucinations. For this reason, it is important for male dentists, hygienists, or assistants to always be escorted by a female assistant when treating women with nitrous oxide. I have been told this is a great distraction from the trauma of having dental care. Men do not seem to have these hallucinations. *We have better control of ourselves.*

In short, nitrous oxide oxygen sedation is very safe for everyone but those with advanced lung disease; heart patients will be safer with this anesthesia than without the gas. It wears off quickly. It is safe and effective for children.

It will work for those who are moderately fearful or who have trouble getting numb.

The problems with pregnancy

At one time, 40% of dentists in America offered nitrous oxide oxygen sedation. The number has fallen some in recent years because not as many dental schools are teaching this technique. There is concern by pregnant staff who work around the trace gas. It has been shown that dental assistants who work around the gas on a daily basis may experience more miscarriages if means are not taken to remove the waste gas from the dental office. There had been no evidence for pregnant patients because they would only use it for an hour or two at the most. Again, we would prefer to not treat pregnant patients. I have taught courses to dentists and dental hygienists since 1969. I have probably given more courses than anyone else in the world only because I started early and have taught for 37 years. The use of nitrous oxide sedation has lowered rather dramatically the number of apprehension patients we see.

What training does a dentist need to do nitrous oxide sedation? A dentist needs either training in dental school or a 14-hour, two-day course that includes practical experience. All dentists should have a Provider Basic Life Support class at least every two years. In addition, many states require those giving nitrous oxide sedation to take an update course every 5-years. No special monitoring is necessary. Patients will always remain awake when using this technique. To the best of my knowledge, there has never been a death using nitrous oxide as a sedative. In fact, you are probably safer using it than not using it because of the added oxygen you are breathing. It was estimated that dentists did close to 80 million cases a year at one time. We are probably down to 10 million a year now.

Oral Conscious Sedation

The next step up in sedation is known as conscious oral sedation or anxiolysis. This is an area of great controversy in dentistry. The American Association of Oral and Maxillofacial surgeons have stated that if a dentist gives even one tablet of a sedative they should be certified to do Intravenous sedation. This simply is not necessary. There is a turf war. The surgeons fear that if general dentists can give oral sedation they may also start extracting wisdom teeth, the major source of income for surgeons.

Oral Conscious Sedation is a level a little beyond what we get with nitrous oxide. You are not as cognitive, will not do well on math tests, but you are not asleep. All your vital reflexes are intact. Your breathing or cardiovascular, heart, is not depressed. In the late 1960s we started to see a class of drugs known as the benzodiazepines (BZDs). The first and probably the best known is Valium, diazepam. The BZDs have replaced the barbiturates and narcotics that were all we had prior to the 1960s. They have an advantage in that their primary action is anti-anxiety. They have little depressant effect on vital reflexes of breathing and heart function. Given alone they are very safe. Later, I will discuss my favorite oral sedative, triazolam, Halcion, a common sleep aid. At one time, something like 7 million prescriptions of this drug were sold every year. Other BZD oral sedatives that work much the same are Ambien, zolpidem, and Xanax, alprazolam.

Oral sedation is safe but slow

Oral medication must be swallowed, it goes first to the stomach and then to the small intestine, where it is absorbed. The lining of the small intestine has enzymes that start breaking down some sedative drugs like the benzodiazepines. It enters the blood stream and goes to the liver where more enzyme is present and more drug is metabolized. Once it leaves the liver it goes to the heart and is pumped to the rest of the body. That goes to the brain, is absorbed, and causes the sedation. This paragraph condensed a subject that can fill whole books.

The problem with all of this is it takes time. To get the effect in the case of triazolam, peak effect is 60 to 90 minutes. The patient takes the pill and you must then wait 60 minutes to start treatment. I think the drug should be administered in the dental office. Everyone reacts differently to medication. A dose that will not affect me may have you close to being asleep. Certainly, the patient should not be left alone after taking the medication; they certainly should not be driving themselves to the office. I strongly believe they should be in the office, take the drug, and be monitored with pulse oximetry, which tells you how much oxygen there is in your blood; blood pressure should be monitored. In addition, the patient should have a dental assistant in the room talking to them just in case they are one of the patients who see greater effect than we expect. That assistant is to keep talking to the patient to assure they do not sleep. If the patient gets close to sleep, the assistant should call the dentist and the drug should be reversed.

Once the patient is relaxed the local anesthesia can be given and the dentistry preformed. This gives us 60 to 90 minutes of working time. The patient is awake but well relaxed. Halcion comes with amnesia. Most patients remember taking the pill and little else until the appointment is over and they are home. A few will remember bits and pieces of the appointment.

Some states require a license to do single agent anxiolysis. I feel the patient should be monitored by taking blood pressures pre sedation and at least every 15 minutes during the sedation. In addition, the patient should be monitored with the use of a pulse oximeter. This monitor measures the percent of oxygen sites on red blood cells that contain an oxygen molecule.

These patients need to come to the dental office an hour early to take their medication and must go home with a responsible adult who will be with them for the next 10 hours. The patient should not make financial decisions, should not be responsible for children or do anything that requires coordination, using power tools, climbing stairs, cooking, or driving for at least 10 hours

There is a reversal agent

Fortunately the BZDs have a reversal agent, Romazicon, Flumazenil. This is important. If a patient becomes a little more sedated than we want, this drug will reverse the sedation within minutes. It is best to give the reversal agent into a vein, but it works almost as fast if injected into the tongue. The dentist needs some training beyond dental school. At least a two-day course or a combination three-day course in nitrous oxide oxygen sedation and oral conscious sedation. In addition, the dentist needs to have had a Provider Basic Life Support course in the last 2 years.

As we start talking about sedation it is imperative that the dentist know your complete medical history and all the drugs you might be on. Some drugs will make the sedatives more potent. Even grapefruit juice has been known to do this.

I had a patient who wanted to be sedated to have a tooth repaired. I looked at his medical history and was a bit wary. I looked at his list of medicines and it was clear he was in heart failure.

I explained I could not sedate him in my office. He would have to go out to the dental school.

I called the dental school and explained I had a difficult patient. They asked me why I did not do him, since I had a good background. I explained I had a perfect record, no deaths in 40 years and, if he died, I would have to practice until I was 105 to get the record back. They said their record, also perfect, was 22 years and they wanted to keep it perfect so they would refer him to the hospital for sedation to be monitored by an anesthesiologist in a setting where there was lots of help in case there was a problem.

There should always be a dental assistant in the room with the patient. This assistant should also be BLS trained. The patient should not leave the office until they can walk with someone holding their arm. These patients should also be with a responsible adult for the next 10 hours.

Deeper oral conscious sedation

The next step is to give more of a single agent or several agents. This may include antihistamines or long acting BZDs, such as xanax. As we give higher doses, the patient may dose off if we do not talk to them or possibly stimulate them by touch to an arm or shoulder. Their breathing and heart function remain unchanged. When we go to this next level where the patient may dose off if not spoken to, the dentist needs a full three day course with additional training on assisting the patients' breathing should they slip into a deeper level of sleep. They also should have some experience in administering IV drugs in case they need to reverse the sedation.

The dentist needs to have had a Provider Basic Life Support course in the last 2 years and preferably an Advanced Cardiac Life Support Course (ACLS). These patients will almost always have amnesia of the whole dental experience. The dentist needs a full three-day course to go to this level of sedation. They need to be taking and recording blood pressures, pulse rates, and oxygen saturation measurements. There should always be a dental assistant in the room with the patient. This assistant should also be BLS trained. They should not leave the office until they can walk with someone holding their arm. These patients should also be with a responsible adult for the next 10 hours.

Intravenous (IV) conscious sedation

The rules are the same as for deeper oral conscious sedation. IV sedation should be safer than oral sedation as you can give a small amount of drug and wait for a minute or two and then add more drug, as needed. It is much easier to titrate, get just the level you need. It is also possible to add a little sedation as the effects starts to wear off.

It is possible, however, to get the patient much deeper than you intended very rapidly. For this reason there are much more stringent requirements of monitoring and education.

Most states require a permit. They require 40 to 60 hours of additional instruction and 20 or more cases of supervised IV sedation. This is an area where, if a dentist does not have good skills or judgment, patients can get into trouble. By definition, the patient remains awake at all times. Because of the nature of the BZD drugs, while the patient is awake they will probably remember nothing of the appointment and even the most phobic patients can be treated safely by a well-trained dentist.

How do you know if your dentist is qualified to go to this level of sedation? First, you want to see their permit. Next, they should have had an Advanced Cardiac Life Support (ACLS) course in the last 2 years. These patients will almost always have amnesia of the whole dental experience. The dentist needs to be taking and recording blood pressures, pulse rates, and oxygen saturation measurements. The dentist and dental assistant should always be in the room with the patient. This assistant should also be BLS trained. The patient should not leave the office until they can walk with someone holding their arm. These patients should also be with a responsible adult for the next 10 hours.

For IV sedation and general anesthesia they will request you have nothing to eat or drink for 8 hours prior to your anesthesia. This is very important if you do not wish to wake up dead. I volunteer every now and again with dental students. We take a couple of dental anesthesiologists and do dentistry of folks who cannot afford care.

A young woman of about 25 needed multiple fillings and some extractions. The anesthesiologist would put her to sleep and I would do the dentistry. They gave her a little drug and asked her if she had had anything to eat that morning. She said no. They gave her a second dose, she went to sleep and I started working. All of a sudden, this bright green hot dog shaped mass came up her throat. I grabbed the suction and started sucking as more and more green goo came up. The anesthesiologist stood laughing, "You have not lost your anesthesia reflexes, Fred."

We woke her up and I told her, "I thought you had nothing to eat this morning." She said, "I was very hungry so we stopped and I had 3 green jelly donuts." We sent her home.

Had I not been on the ball with the suction and had she inhaled the green goo she could have died. If you are going to be sedated, follow orders. We require you to do these things for your safety.

She was back a month later, same directions, nothing to eat or drink. As she came into the clinic, she was sucking on an extra tall coffee. Some people just want to die.

Deep IV sedation / general anesthesia

We are now in the big leagues. The patient will be in and out of consciousness or completely unconscious. They will remember nothing of the appointment. The dentist will usually use local anesthesia for pain control and use the sedation/general anesthesia to keep the patient comfortable. The dentist needs to be fully trained. This would require a full anesthesia residency. Thirty five years ago that meant a one-year residency. In the 2000s it is a 2-year full time residency in a hospital or a dental school. An oral surgeon can qualify if they have had a fully-certified oral surgery residency. This residency usually includes 3 to 6 months of doing general anesthesia in a hospital operating room and some time doing out-patient anesthesia in a surgery clinic.

Why do I think a separate anesthesiologist is needed? I volunteer to do dentistry in a clinic where underprivileged patients are treated. We had very uncooperative 5 year old with decay in most of his teeth. It simply was not possible to treat him awake and we could not wait as some of his teeth were already infected and needed to be extracted. I was tagged to do the dentistry because of my anesthesia background.

There would be a dental anesthesiologist who would do the anesthesia. The child was sedated in the hall. He was brought into the treatment room, and the dental anesthesiologist started an IV. Monitors were applied and he was put to sleep being monitored by the anesthesiologist.

I started to work doing his fillings. He developed a laryngeal spasm, and his vocal cords spasmed shut. This is a fairly common anesthesia complication and was handled promptly and correctly by the dental anesthesiologist. At this point, the boy developed a bronchial spasm where the small air tubes in his lungs went into spasm and closed down.

This spasm prevented the anesthesiologist from breathing effectively for him. A second anesthesiologist came to help. The two anesthesiologists worked for an hour before they controlled and reversed the problem.

The boy survived with no ill effects. However, for about 45 minutes, I feared he would die. The two anesthesiologists declared their day was done at 2PM. They were exhausted. Had they not both been there, I fear the outcome would have been different.

Would this child have survived had a dental assistant been left with him. What do you think?

Would I let a dentist or surgeon put me to sleep if they were not a fully trained anesthesiologist, even one who had a full one or two year residency? In a word, no – not a snowball's chance in hell.

Certification

There is one other certifying agency. The American Society of Dental Anesthesiology has a board that requires a full residency. This is the American Board of Dental Anesthesiology. There is one other organization that at one time required a full anesthesia residency but now has dentists who have not had full residencies. This is the American Dental Society of Anesthesiology and its National Board of Dental Anesthesiology. While most members have had a full one-year residency not all of them are so trained. I would not accept the Fellowship of the American Dental Society of Anesthesiology, FADSA, as proof of adequate training.

There have been deaths

Is it really necessary to have a full two-year residency to give general anesthesia? Yes. Anesthesia is defined as great amounts of boredom disbursed with moments of stark terror. In a two year residency, the dentists will have seen such moments and will understand how severe the outcome can be if everything is not done right. In 2003, there were 2 deaths from anesthesia/surgery complications in dentistry in the state of Washington. One death was the second for one of the surgeons. Nationwide I heard of 8 other deaths. The American Association of Maxillofacial Surgeons admits in self-reported studies that their members see one death for every 700,000 anesthetics. That is a very good record unless you are the one who dies. In that case it is 100%.

Is it safe to give anesthesia and do dentistry?

There are some who question if it is safe to give the anesthetic and do the surgery / dentistry. There was a study in the United Kingdom in the 1970 that showed the death rate was twice as high if the dentist was both the anesthesiologist and the surgeon. We do have better monitors now; but we have no studies to show that it is any safer to do both. The surgeon / dentist should be in the room full time from the time the patient is put to sleep until he is awake. At no time should the surgeon who is giving the anesthesia leave to numb up in a different room, remove teeth in a different room leaving the patient under general anesthesia with either a dental assistant or registered nurse. A possible exception would be a Certified Registered Nurse Anesthetist.

When do we do what

When are the various modalities of pain control indicated? Always start with local anesthesia. Nitrous oxide can be added with no increase in risk. The next step to anxiolysis, light conscious oral sedation, is equally safe. As we go to more profound sedation the training and risk go up. Even general anesthesia is quite safe if a separate dental or medical anesthesiologist gives the anesthesia. Some surgical procedures require general anesthesia because it is not possible to get a patient completely numb with local anesthesia.

Rules for me

I personally would not let the same person give me anesthesia who is going to do the surgery. They do not do it in medicine; I do not think we should do it in dentistry. What really concerns me is the office that leaves a patient under deep sedation with a dental assistant or even a registered nurse while the dentist goes to a different area of the office to start or finish another case. This is commonly done in some surgery offices.

General anesthesia is known to have some risks. That's why it is imperative that you tell the person giving you anesthesia about any medical problems you have and all medications you might be taking; even over the counter and natural remedies are important.

> *There was a patient who went to an oral surgeon to have 5 teeth removed. She told the surgeon she had airway problems when they operated on her hips. They had to wake her up and do a tracheotomy to be able to breathe for her. She showed the dentist the scar.*

> *The surgeon put her to sleep and was unable to breathe for her. After about 5 minutes without breathing she had a heart attack and died despite the surgeon and EMTs' best efforts to resuscitate her. It turned out she also had some undiagnosed heart problems. Had she had a strong heart she might have lived 10 minutes. However, her airway problems should have been a red flag to the dentist, saying, "do not put me to sleep." It is your life. If you have had anesthesia problems in the past, first find out whether you really do have to be asleep, and if so, you should be in a hospital.*

How about emergency preparedness? I have seen dental office emergency kits with drugs that were 25 years old. Another one had drugs so old the clear fluids were picking up the color of the stoppers in their cartridges. Does your dentist have an automatic external defibrillator, AED?

Florida passed regulations requiring all dental offices to have AEDs, automatic external defibrillators as of February 2006. These devices are automatic and can shock a fibrillating heart back into a normal rhythm. Without this shock, the survival rate of patients with heart ventricular fibrillation drops 10% each minute waiting for the EMTs to come with their defibrillator. Defibrillators are found in sports arenas, airports, hotels, and even on most commercial aircraft. I think they should also be in dental offices. They are imperative if IV sedation or general anesthesia are being done.

 Ask your dentist. If they have one in their office you know they take emergency preparedness seriously. If you are going to have IV sedation or general anesthesia I would insist on it.

I use the "Me Test" would I want me to be put to sleep in those surroundings, by someone with that training? I would insist on a dentist or medical anesthesiologist who has had a full anesthesia residency to put me to sleep and monitor me full time while I was under anesthesia. I would not be put to sleep by the same person who was doing the surgery or dentistry. Remember dead is for a very long time.

V. Mainline dentistry

HERMAN®

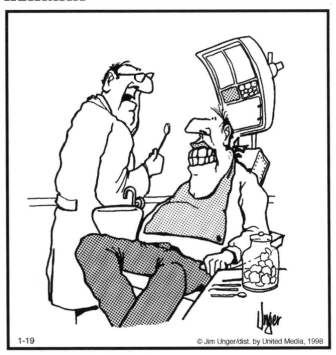

1-19 © Jim Unger/dist. by United Media, 1998

**"It'll take you a couple of days
to get used to them."**

12. Restorative Dentistry – fillings

You can be ugly the rest of your life with silver, or beautiful for the next 10 years with tooth colored fillings.

Why are fillings done?

When part of a tooth is lost due to decay or chipping it should be replaced. If a hole is left, bacteria and food can lodge in this area and cause further loss of structure. This sounds very simple.

There are two basic forms of decay, smooth surface decay and groove decay. The smooth surface decay forms on the buccal (front) or lingual (back) surfaces of the teeth. They can also form on the surfaces of the teeth where they touch the adjacent tooth in the arch. You do not immediately get a hole on these surfaces. First, calcium is removed from the structure; however, a matrix of tooth structure still exists. The surface and underlying enamel takes on a chalky white appearance and is softer than sound tooth. It is a bit like Swiss cheese except the holes are on a microscopic level. A percentage of the Calcium of the tooth has been leached from the sound tooth structure. At this level of destruction it is possible to remineralize the defect.

Remineralizing early decay

Remineralization is a process of driving calcium ions back into the tooth to replace those that have been lost. With daily fluoride use, it is possible to remineralize decay that has taken calcium from the enamel well into the softer dentin of the tooth. It may take a few years but it can be done. There have been some toothpastes sold that were reported to do the same. Certainly fluoride tooth pastes helped prevent decay and may remineralize very early decay.

Using a fluoride gel

The best way to remineralize is with a fluoride gel. Fluoride is available over the counter in most states at a 1/2 percent concentration. This is much more concentrated than you find in toothpaste and previously available fluoride mouth rinses that were 1/20%.

Xylitol

There is some evidence that if you use xylitol, a sugar, you can do the same. Why not just use some fluoride and xylitol every day just in case you have unknown areas of decay? This is a very good idea. If this were done you would have a very low chance of ever getting decay. Even if there is decay evident in x-rays it is highly likely that it can be remineralized.

Groove decay

Decay in grooves may be a different matter. There is some controversy here. Some dentists believe if there is even stain in grooves they should be filled. This assumes that the person is not a smoker. Smoking will stain even normal grooves. I have seen many patients who lose teeth at 70 or 80 years old. They have stain in grooves that did not have decay. I have sectioned some of these teeth and found very small inactive areas of decay in the bottom of the groove. These might have been a problem by the time they were 120 years old.

What is the correct indication to do a filling in a groove? We clearly do not know. My opinion and what I would do in my own mouth is as follows: if an explorer, pick, sticks in the groove, I would fill it. If the groove is stained but has no stick I would not fill it. It is possible that one of these groove decays would continue to get deeper and eventually involve the nerve of the tooth. I have seen that happen maybe 3 times in 40 years. If you get your teeth checked every 6 months and use fluoride the chance is very small, however.

Once there is decay in a tooth, part of the tooth structure is gone. There is a hole. In addition to looking bad, these areas are full of bacteria and food that cause the decay to progress making the hole get larger and larger. The bacteria will eventually reach the nerve or pulp of the tooth. Once this happens the tooth will need endodontic treatment or it will need to be extracted.

The filling process

The process of placing a filling starts with numbing the tooth and then removing the soft decayed structure. Once all the decay is removed, the preparation (prep for short) must be done. We have to make the prep in a shape that is appropriate for the material we will use to replace the missing structure. We will also remove any undermined structure, areas of the tooth that are vulnerable to future decay and possibly some sound tooth structure to make it possible to place the filling.

What material can we use?

When we chew we have the small points, cusps, of our teeth contact the teeth in the opposite arch. Most folks can bite down with a force of around 100 pounds. The contact points may be as small as 0.5 to 0.25 sq.mm. in area. This results in loads of up to 40,000 pounds per square inch. It takes a very strong material to take loads of this magnitude.

What is an ideal filling material? We want a material that looks like tooth, is low cost, easy to manipulate, sets up as hard as tooth enamel, bonds to the enamel, and will not let bacteria invade the microscopic space between the filling material and the tooth. No such material exists.

Materials, silver amalgam, gold, or composite – direct or indirect

There are three basic groups of materials, silver amalgam, gold, and tooth colored material composites. These may be direct fillings, formed within the tooth, or indirect.

Indirect fillings

Indirect restorations are made by preparing a hole in the tooth that removes the decay and tapers slightly to the occlusal (top) surface of the tooth. An impression material is squirted into the preparation and makes a mold of the preparation and the rest of the tooth. A temporary filling is then placed in the hole.

The impression is sent to a dental lab that forms a material in a very accurate model of the tooth. This material is then sent back to the dentist who cements it into the preparation at a second appointment.

Silver amalgam and gold

Silver amalgam and gold have been the standard for years. Gold came first and silver amalgam next. There was great controversy when silver amalgam first became available. It split the dental association into two very opposed groups and was known as the amalgam wars.

Gold fillings

Gold fillings are the benchmark. They are the finest, most long-lasting material we have. Gold fillings are 5 to 7 times more expensive than silver fillings but lest costly than indirect tooth colored fillings. If well done they can last a life time. If poorly done, they will fail in a year or two.

Gold foil

There is also a direct gold restoration. A direct restoration is formed in the tooth rather than in the laboratory. Gold foil is done by taking small balls of pure gold foil and tapping them into very small preparations. Pure gold will weld to itself when compressed. In this way a solid piece of gold can be formed inside a very conservative small preparation. These are very difficult, time-consuming restorations; consequently, they are very costly. Since the advent of tooth colored bonded materials, gold fillings are rarely done.

Gold inlays and onlays

There are several classes of gold fillings. Inlays fit within the cusps and replace the area of the tooth lost to decay. Onlays are like an inlay but extend over one or more cusps. By shoeing (covering the cusp) the tooth is protected from splitting. These require one appointment to prepare the tooth, take an impression to send to the lab, and have a temporary filling placed. The gold restoration is cemented at a second appointment. Their cost has less to do with the cost of gold than the time spent by the dentist and the lab in preparing the tooth, fabricating the gold fillings and cementing it in the mouth. They are the most durable of any of our materials.

Unfortunately, gold is not tooth colored. If it were this would be the hands down winner of the filling choices. Their biggest disadvantage is their gold color. They just do not look like teeth. The other issue is their cost. While they do last longer than silver filings they do not last 7 times longer. If you can ignore the cost and if they are well done, they are the most durable restoration your dentist can do.

Silver fillings

Silver fillings are only partly made of silver. They are more properly called a silver amalgam filling. An amalgam is an alloy of mercury and some other metal. What does this all mean? After the tooth is prepared, a powder comprised of filings of a silver, tin, copper, and zinc alloy is mixed with about an equal amount of mercury. The mercury dissolves the outer surface of the metal filings. This outer surface contacts the outer surface of other particles and recrystalizes into a new metal alloy of silver, tin, copper, zinc, and mercury. This bonds all the filings together in one very strong mass.

It takes about four hours for the mix to set up hard enough to accept chewing loads without breaking. The material continues to harden for about a week. You should not worry about chewing if you wait out the first four hours, however.

Silver amalgam is brittle

The material is brittle. As it is exposed to chewing forces, over the years the margins where the metal touches the tooth will chip. This is not a problem so long as the chipping is small, less than 0.5 mm, the thickness of 3 or 4 pieces of paper. The worry has been that once these small imperfections form, decay and saliva can "leak" between the tooth and silver and get to the inner softer dentin of the tooth.

Do silver fillings leak

For years we looked at the gray halo in the enamel of teeth with old fillings and said they leaked and should be replaced. We now know this does not happen. The silver in the small defects will corrode and seal the space preventing bacteria from migrating to the inner structures. If the defect is bigger you can get decay at the base of the chip. How do I decide if a filling needs to be replaced? If the chip is large enough to trap food, is soft or greater then 1 mm wide, I replace it or just repair that chip. How can you tell? If you can feel the catch with your fingernail in the groove the time has probably come.

Watch out for the intraoral camera shot

Some dentists will take an intraoral camera and enlarge the image of the tooth many times on a TV monitor. It really looks bad, but remember it is 50 times normal size. If the dentist is doing this and telling you how corroded the filling is I would be a little suspicious. The best silver fillings are beat up, stained, and chipped but have no soft tooth structure next to the alloy indicating there is decay. They got that way by chewing for many years. If they have not broken, they will probably be around many more years if we are smart enough to leave them alone.

Should alloy be polished?

Alloy, in various forms, has been used in dentistry for at least 200 years. Its biggest disadvantage is its appearance. The color varies from bright shiny silver to black, depending on how well the patient cleans it and if it was polished. There is no evidence that polished alloy lasts better then unpolished. It cannot be polished for at least a day after it is placed because it is too soft the first day.

Silver is the least costly, most durable material we have

The biggest advantage of silver fillings is their cost. It is much less costly than any other material we use. Not only is the material less costly it is easy to place so the cost of these restorations is the least costly of any other material. It also lasts very well. I have placed many alloy fillings that are still serving 25 years after they were placed. It is by far the most cost effective material we have. You get more chews per buck than with any other material.

I thought mercury was poison

The silver amalgam filling is 50% mercury. Mercury comes in several forms; elemental mercury is the silver metal, a liquid at room temperature, of thermometers. While it is toxic, we should not drink it or play with it, it is of no risk once it is in a filling.

The mad hatter of *Alice in Wonderland* was probably mad because as a hat maker he cured the beaver pelts used for hats with mercury compounds. His exposure as a hatter was a problem. In the early days of dentistry, dentists would squeeze the excess mercury out of filling materials by placing it in a cloth and squeezing with his (there were very few women dentists in those days) bare hands. This was before we used rubber gloves. This practice led to excessive exposure for dentists and some reports of mercury toxicity for dentists.

Organic mercury is very toxic

The ionic form of mercury is very toxic. Methylmercury is very toxic. We had a swimming pool at one time. When it warmed up in the summer we had a major problem with black spots forming on the sides of the pool. The pool maintenance companies sold us a chemical mixture that was great for killing the fungus causing these spots. This chemical disappeared from the market. When I asked why, I was told because it was a mercury compound. It sure worked well against the fungus, however.

There was a bay in Japan that had a factory that discharged these ionic mercury compounds into the bay. The members of a village of Minamata Japan, on the shore of this bay depended on fish from this bay for food. Because of the high levels of ionic mercury waste in the bay, many children were born to the villagers that were severely retarded. Organic mercury is very bad stuff.

This problem with the toxic forms of mercury surfaced in a toxic antifungal of organic mercury. This compound was used on seed grains and worked well, but when humans consumed these seeds there were tragic consequences. Often these seeds were colored pink to indicate they were only for planting. During the early 1970s there was a severe drought in Iraq. People facing starvation could not read the warnings on the bags. The pink grain made bread toxic. Many people died or were disabled. There have been other outbreaks of poisoning due to organic mercury compounds.

As children, when we had cuts or scrapes, we were painted with Mercurochrome or Merthiolate. These were bright orange red. Some kids called it monkey blood. It was obvious to all that you had a wound. It was used as a disinfectant. When we got sore throats our throats were painted with the medicaments. I do not know if it worked but it tasted bad and hurt when it was being painted on the back of our throats. We quickly learned to not tell our mothers if we had a sore throat. She was sure it helped us heal and prevented sore throats. We never told her we would die before we would admit to a sore throat and the throat painting.

These were a form of mercury. It is a compound merbromin or dibromohydroxymercurifluoriscein disodium salt. With a name like that, it has to be effective. It probably was a bit toxic. It did kill bacteria. However, other than a few ticks and twitches, I seem to have survived these medications. They have been banned in the US but are available in many parts of the world.

Elemental mercury is not very toxic

The elemental form of mercury does not change to the ionic form without heating it to very high levels, over 400 degrees. There is no risk of it forming the methyl-mercury from our silver fillings. It has been stated that if you eat two tuna fish or salmon meals a year, you get more mercury from your fish than you do from a mouth full of fillings. The larger fish eat smaller fish that eat smaller fish that eat plankton that filter seawater that has miniscule levels of mercury. Each predator level concentrates those chemicals found in the lower level predators. By the time you get to the largest fish there are very low levels of mercury but the level is higher than what you get from your silver fillings.

Elemental mercury is, in fact, natural. Our mountains of the Northwest have cinnabar deposits; the ore mercury is refined from. Our streams and rivers have been flushing mercury into our sounds since the last ice age. In fact, nature is by far the largest contributor of mercury to the environment.

Some dentists will suggest silver fillings are dangerous

Some dentists whose ethics are a bit elastic recount these problems to their patients as a reason to have all their silver fillings removed and replaced with composite and porcelain fillings at great cost. These composite and porcelain fillings simply do not last very well. A well-done alloy filling may last 25 years or more. The average composite filling is lucky to last 10 or 12 years. The cast porcelain fillings, I will discuss later, will last until you bite hard enough to break them. Often that is within a year or two.

> *WASHINGTON—A U.S. federal appeals court said Friday, March 13, 2007, it could not force the Food and Drug Administration to tighten restrictions on dental fillings containing mercury.*
>
> *Advocacy groups sought to ban the use of such fillings and to force the FDA to classify them as risky, subjecting them to tougher regulations.*
> *The mercury mixture has stirred controversy since dentists began using it to fill cavities in the 1800s. Significant levels of mercury exposure can cause permanent damage to the brain and kidneys, but the FDA has said for years that mercury fillings don't harm patients, except in rare cases when they have allergic reactions.*

Consumer Reports take on silver fillings

The *Consumer Reports* magazine in the 1980s reported on the issue of replacing alloy fillings.

They made a statement that went something like this. The best reason to replace a patient's silver fillings is fluoride. I read that statement and thought this made no sense. What does fluoride have to do with silver fillings? I read the next paragraph and it was made clear. They went on to state that because of fluoride in our toothpastes, and water, there is much less decay to fill. This leaves a cavity in the wallets of many dentists. To fill that cavity they were removing silver fillings and replacing them with composite fillings. Now it was clear.

At least one dentist was prosecuted, lost his license, and was given jail time for telling people that their diseases, everything from Muscular Dystrophy to forgetfulness and amnesia, were caused by their silver fillings. He wrote books and is still occasionally seen on TV talk shows. He would remove your silver and go through other treatments to remove the mercury from your system. Others dentists and other health care practitioners have suggested everything from special drinks to enemas to remove the mercury from our bodies. I guess that is really cleansing the body from both ends.

Is the mercury a problem for dentists

There have been several studies of dentists since we work around mercury all the time to see if we are absorbing mercury. I have been involved in two such studies. Both times I came out with levels below that of persons not exposed to mercury. There are machines that are sensitive enough to measure the level of mercury vapor in a patient's mouth after they have chewed. Should this be a concern? Probably not, they measure levels in parts per billion.

Amalgam cannot be flushed down the sewer

There has been a whole industry develop opposed to amalgam. I have had to add traps to my waste lines to keep silver filings that come from people's teeth from entering the sewer system. There is no science that I am doing any harm. In fact, the level in the waste stream is 1/100 of what federal guidelines allow. I would have to do 100 times as many silver fillings as I now do, work 24 hours a day, 7 days a week with 30 dentists to approach that level in my sewer. Of course none of the patients or the staff could have a bowel movement while in the office as that would dilute the levels of mercury in our sewer out flow. Are we being a little silly?

I like amalgam fillings

Why am I so pro silver filling? It allows me to provide dental care to a lot of patients at a lower price than any other material available. It lasts better than other materials. It has been estimated that if you consider the longevity of composite fillings as opposed to silver fillings and the difference in cost, composite fillings cost 3 times more per chew than silver fillings.

I have been told there is a conspiracy to keep me using silver. I do not know who is directing that conspiracy. If I am being pressured or duped, it is very subtle as I am not aware of the pressure. It is to me a simple matter of economics. Silver lasts longer and is less costly for my patients. The best thing that could happen to me from a business sense is to have silver outlawed. I would have to work 7 days a week, 24 hours a day to replace all the silver in people's mouths and I would have a guaranteed business as the composite fillings will break down and need to replaced far more often. From a business standpoint I should be leading the attack on silver.

Has amalgam been banned?

There have been a few patients reported to be allergic to this material and with those exceptions, no one has ever been harmed by silver fillings. It is a good material and should continue to be used. However, at the rate we are going it could be outlawed. You will hear that it has been outlawed in Scandinavia and Canada. At this writing neither is true. We are seeing many moves to outlaw us from putting it into the sewer systems as we take failing fillings out of patient's teeth. I have even heard that undertakers are having problems because of the mercury vapor that is released when a body is cremated. I feel comfortable enough about this material that every member of my family has silver fillings.

The choice is yours – silver, gold, or composite

Having said all of the above. If you want your silver fillings removed and replaced with composite fillings, I will agree, provided you listen to my explanation that it is not necessary from a health basis and that the composite fillings will not last as long and are more expensive. It is your mouth and it is your right to have tooth colored fillings if you want them. It is also your right to believe that the silver is detrimental to you health and that it should be removed. So long as you understand I do not agree with that belief, I will honor your wish. It is OK to have fillings that are tooth colored so long as I have explained the advantages and disadvantages of such fillings.

As an insurance consultant I have seen many excuses used to try to justify removing alloy fillings and changing them to tooth colored fillings. In general, most insurances cover the least costly professionally accepted material. Silver clearly wins. One of the most inventive reasons to change came from a dentist who wanted to remove 5 silver fillings and replace them with porcelain fillings. Total cost for the change, $4,000. He stated, "I saw Mrs. X. She is a healthy 54 year old who has buzzing coming from her fillings. Scientifically, this phenomenon has been shown to occur with silver fillings. The only cure is to remove the silver and replace them with porcelain fillings." The dentist and patient can agree to this change but it is not covered under any insurance policy that I am aware of.

My response after denying coverage was, "whatever you do, do not remove the silver restorations. Have you evaluated the buzzing for frequency shift or pulsation? With proper cryptographic analysis we might find an embedded message. If you remove the fillings, mankind will for all time lose this channel of communication with the great beyond." My secretary brought the letter to me and said we could not send the letter, and said it was stupid. I responded, "it is not as stupid as what the dentist wrote." She refused to send the letter so instead, we suggested he refer the patient to an ear specialist and the dentist to a psychiatrist.

Tooth-colored fillings

Porcelain had been the generic name for tooth colored materials. In fact very few fillings were truly porcelain. When I was in dental school, we all did a porcelain inlay. They only worked on the smallest areas of decay that were not placed in areas of stress. A few were probably done for areas of stress but very few practitioners were able to do these and have success.

Most fillings that were done were either silicate or plastic materials. The silicate fillings dissolved and had to be redone every few years. The plastic developed a dark brown to black line around the filling within a year. They were also very soft. They lasted better than silicate but were ugly.

Direct composite fillings

The tooth colored materials are direct or indirect depending on whether the filling material is formed at the lab or in the mouth. They are further classified as to whether they are a composite or porcelain. In the late 1970s, we started to see composite fillings. These are basically a plastic material mixed with very small particals of hard materials, crystals of some salts or porcelain.

The composite sets when exposed to a bright light

These materials are squirted into the prep, and a bright light is directed to the material that causes it to set nearly as hard as tooth structure. Depending on the strength of the light, this can take only seconds.

Prior to these materials, all fillings were either held in place by undercuts and dovetails or cemented in place. The modern composites are as strong as tooth, have great color, and bond to the underlying tooth. These can actually strengthen badly broken down teeth. The color of these if matched carefully can be impossible to tell from tooth.

They are difficult to do well

They are difficult to do, take many steps, and once they are set, they are very hard and difficult to shape to a tooth form. For all of these reasons they are more costly than silver fillings. Some say they should be twice as expensive. They usually are at least 50% more costly because of the additional time it takes to place them. If there is a marginal defect, either an incomplete fill or a poor bond, these will not seal like an alloy. I have seen requests to replace these only a few years after they were placed because of new decay at the margins.

Indirect fillings

The next advancement in restorative material was indirect restorations. These can be of composite or porcelain materials. The indirect restorations are formed from a model of the tooth. After the tooth is prepared an impression is made with a silicon or rubber material. A temporary is then placed in the tooth and the patient is sent home for a week or two.

This impression has very hard plaster poured into the mold. Once the plaster sets, it is removed and is a very accurate model of the tooth and the preparation that was made. The restoration is then formed in the lab on this model. This is much easier than doing them directly in the mouth. Because of this, the appearance of these can be spectacular. However, the lab charge for this service increases the cost of the restoration about $200 to $300.

Indirect composites are expensive

The patient comes back after the restoration has been fabricated and it is bonded in place. The cost of the restoration is often over $1,000 in metropolitan areas. The porcelain or composite can not be made with the accuracy of a gold inlay. If the fit has a gap of less then 200 micron, 0.2 mm—about the thickness of a piece of paper, it is considered adequate and is bonded in place with a type of composite.

These indirect restorations are very costly, probably 5-7 times greater than a similar amalgam, silver, and filling. They do not fit very well. They are about 60% as strong as a tooth. So you can pay 7 times more than an alloy for a filling that is weak. Why do dentists suggest this and why do patients pay for them? In a word, aesthetics.

My dentist no longer does silver fillings

It has almost become a badge of honor for a dentist to say, "I no longer do silver fillings. I am an aesthetic dentist. I do quality dentistry." What is not said is, "I can make more money, I can charge more, and I only have to work with the rich folks who are more like me." (Please see the section on quality dentistry.)

To attract people that can and will afford this service it is necessary to practice in affluent areas. It is usually necessary to market the service and to stretch the truth a little about the benefits of the porcelain fillings. It is often necessary to play to the emotions of the patient. This will make you more beautiful, accepted, and successful. Some take the approach, if you really are successful you will be able to afford this treatment. We will remove those poisonous fillings and replace them with our holistic materials.

Direct restorations can be made from a variety materials. Typically, super strong composites much like the materials used for direct fillings are formed under pressure and heat on the tooth model to make a harder composite than is possible with a direct restoration that is formed in the mouth. These are weaker and tend to wear faster than the true porcelain fillings or tooth.

Other porcelain options

Other indirect restorations are various forms of porcelain, some very strong, others somewhat weaker. These are basically fused glass that has coloring to match the color of the tooth. The weaker ones tend to have a little better color.

Computer formed fillings

One system uses an image taken with an optical probe. No impression is necessary. This image is sent to a milling machine that forms the restoration from a solid block of porcelain by grinding away the unwanted material. These do not look quite as nice as the block is one color. They do not fit as well, as the machine is not as accurate as other systems. They are completed the same day, however. They tend to be more costly than the two appointment porcelain restorations because the optical probe and the milling machine cost well over $100,000. You must do a lot of these to pay for the machine much less make a profit. It probably takes about 500 restorations to justify the cost of the machine as compared to sending the impression to a lab and having a porcelain restoration fabricated.

You have many complex choices

Did you ever believe your choices could be so complex? I have sat through whole day lectures on the indirect porcelain fillings. It took a second day to get information on the direct fillings. There are so many different materials, even classes of materials, that it is very difficult to know what material is best for which situation. It often comes down to the material the dentist's lab uses. As one lecturer stated, "You can have an ugly silver filling for most of your life or a tooth-colored one for 10 years. It is your choice."

If you come away from this chapter with the opinion that silver fillings are very safe and serve very well at a modest cost, I have been successful. Tooth-colored fillings are more costly, too much more costly, but can restore a tooth to its natural form and color; however, they will wear faster and break more often and not last as long. If you understand all of this, I have done my job.

When to fill

It can be very difficult to decide at what point the groove of a tooth needs a filling. There is no consensus among dentists as to just when it should be filled. The old standard was to push an explorer into a groove; if it stuck, it was time to fill, but this test is not accepted by all dentists.

Some think you should fill if there is stain in the groove. Others feel you need a laser detector to decide. Even these dentists have not decided at what reading on this laser a tooth should be filled.

Some decay can be reversed

Smooth surfaces of teeth are not easier to decide on the point of filling unless there is a hole. Demineralization, that chalky white decay, can and should be remineralized. Fluoride has been shown to be very effective in doing this. Fluoride is now available over the counter in gels that can reverse these early areas of decay. Fluoride in our water systems has helped remineralize and strengthen tooth structures preventing much of the smooth surface decay we once saw.

You must do your part

Because of the difficulty of knowing when decay has progressed to a level that needs restoration, having a checkup every 6 to 9 months makes sense, particularly if you see any initial signs of decay, chalkiness, early x-ray signs or stain in any grooves. If you are willing to do your part by brushing and flossing and using daily fluorides, many of these are will never progress and some may even remineralize and never need restorations.

The filling is not the end

Once a tooth has a filling, it will need to be filled again and again throughout life. Each replacement will be a bit larger and if you start early enough with decay and live long enough, many of these teeth will eventually need crowns. Even crowns are not the end of the line as they need to be redone in time. It is best to not get decay or to remineralize the decay if you get behind and develop early small areas. Once there is a hole, you have no choice but to repair the defect.

HERMAN®

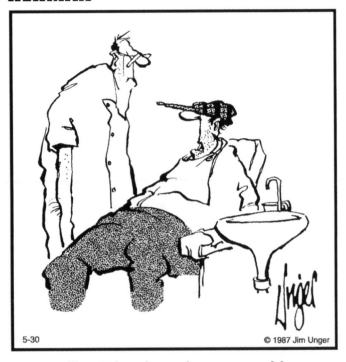

5-30
© 1987 Jim Unger

**"Last time I was here you said
I probably needed a cap."**

When do you need a crown / cap

If a tooth is badly broken down, is missing one
of its cusps, it may need a crown, or cap. Many
believe all back teeth with root canals need
crowns as these teeth are prone to breakage.
Most do not believe this is necessary for front
teeth with root canals unless the tooth is badly
broken down. The crown surrounds the tooth

holding the tooth together and making it as strong as possible. Crowns are also used to makeover badly stained teeth or teeth that are out of position, where a veneer will not work. This falls into the area of dentistry being done for aesthetics vs. for strength.

Crowns come in a variety of forms

Stainless steel crowns

We use stainless steel shells to build up teeth in children. These are 1/3 the cost of a regular crown. These shells come in a variety of sizes and shapes. They are cut and crimped to fit as well as possible. If they are placed on a primary (baby) tooth that has to last 5 years, they work well. I have also used them on adults where the patient could not afford a conventional crown. Some of these have lasted 25 years. I worry, however, because they fit a little like a washtub on a fence post. They certainly are irritating to the gum tissue. However, some patients have saved teeth this way that might otherwise have been lost.

Gold crowns

Gold crowns were the standard. Why gold? It wears about the same as tooth. It does not tend to wear opposing teeth. It can be made to fit very accurately, is easy to adjust and polish, is strong, and it works. However, it does not look like a white tooth.

Porcelain and metal crowns

Porcelain and metal, PFM, porcelain fused to metal crowns have a metal thimble that fits over the tooth. This is usually an alloy of gold that has had other metals added to it to make it melt at a higher temperature than gold. Some of the metals are non precious. Some patients will have allergic reactions to these non precious metals. Porcelain is then fired to the metal thimble in the form and color of the tooth being repaired. Porcelain fuses at close to 1800 degrees and gold melts at a little over 1800 degrees. The metals used for these crowns melt at over 2600 degrees so they can stand up to the heat necessary to add porcelain.

These crowns are 50% stronger than natural teeth. They are very hard and will wear opposing teeth and gold crowns. They look very good. If well done, they can be impossible to tell from natural teeth. However, they are not quite as aesthetic as the all porcelain crowns.

All Porcelain Crown

These are all porcelain, no metal. They can be beautiful, if well done. They have natural translucency not seen in any other material. However, they vary between 60% to 90% as strong as natural teeth. In a patient with very light teeth, these may be the only way to get a good match. So it can be perfect but it will not be quite as strong.

What about missing teeth

When a tooth is lost, in general with a few exceptions, it should be replaced. If it is not replaced remaining teeth may shift, food traps may form, gum damage may result. Will you die of this? No. But it still is better to replace missing teeth. We now can do this with implants. There are places where a bridge makes more sense.

How is a bridge done?

To do a bridge, you prep the teeth on either side of the space and put a crown on these teeth. The two teeth are joined by a fake tooth attached to both of the crowns. So you essentially have three teeth as one unit. The two end crowns are called abutments. The fake tooth in between is called a pontic. This is all cemented in place as one unit.

When is the bridge the best option?

When does it make since to do a bridge rather than an implant? If adjacent teeth have large decay, large fillings that will have to be replaced eventually, have shifted, have had root canals, it makes sense to crown these as part of a bridge. In this case, the cost of the bridge is that of three crowns

When should an implant with a crown be placed?

If the adjacent teeth are virgin, have never had decay, fillings or have small fillings, have not had root canals, are pristine, I really do not like to cut them down for crowns. In makes more sense to do an implant and then place a crown over the implant post. This is about 30% more costly than a bridge. There is evidence that is slowly emerging that implants may well outlast bridges.

This has been a far too long discussion of the materials and techniques used to repair teeth. But it does serve to show just how many options you have.

13. The miracle smile makeover

America is the culture of deception when it comes to our appearance. Wigs, hairpieces, hair implants, electrolysis, body shapers, teeth the color of Chiclets, toilet bowl white, and fake boobs.

Even our pets are not immune. We have teeth whitening toothpaste for dogs, and neuticles to replace the testicles removed when we neuter our dogs and cats, or even horses and bulls.

Over the last decade TV has shown many cases where various patients had plastic surgery, stomach stapling, and a number of other procedures to correct various imperfections— everything from big ears and disfigured noses through surgical help to lose massive amounts of weight, and smile makeovers. We are expected to look in awe at the freshly minted beauty, and in many cases the results are nice. But did you ever wonder what happens to these patients after some time passes?

Some makeover aspects are long lasting, others are not. But let's focus on dental makeovers now. People think of such a makeover the way they think of visiting the hair salon. But a dental makeover should be considered much more carefully. The difference between a miracle smile makeover and a new haircut is that your hair will grow back but the enamel of your teeth once removed is gone forever.

Realize as you read this chapter that there are reasons to do smile makeovers. If you smile in the mirror every morning and hate yourself because of your smile, you can change it. If your dentures are loose so that you cannot chew with them, there are solutions. Be sure, however, that a dental makeover is your own idea, and not that of a fast-talking smile designer. Be particularly sure that the dentistry you get done is age appropriate. For example, you probably do not need a smile makeover for your 90th birthday. And if you have a smile make over in your 20s, realize that you will need to have it redone many times in your life and there might come a time when you lose many teeth because of what was done in your 20s. Be sure you have all the facts before starting down this street.

People pay hundreds if not thousands of dollars on their appearance. From the latest clothes and accessories, to hairdressers, and makeup artists. The wealthy spend more on such care than I can imagine.

What is so terrible to take a similar amount of money and spend it on the "perfect smile?" The big difference is you can give away the clothes and accessories and purchase the latest style when you tire of these. All you have done is disposed of some of your disposable income. That same can be said about the cost of the hairdresser and makeup artists. The makeup can be washed off and done again. That hair will regrow with time.

When you start trimming gingival, gum, tissue and cutting down teeth, it is forever. The loss of structure will, for all time, leave those teeth weaker. It cannot be regrown. The crowns, veneers, will, in time, need to be redone. More tooth will be taken and the remaining structure will be weaker. The trauma to the teeth may eventually cause the pulp to die necessitating a root canal, endodontic treatment.

These smile makeovers are not forever unless you consider having to be redone periodically for the rest of your life forever or if you step off the curb in front of a truck.

An extreme dental patient

One patient who has been featured on several TV shows started at close to 500 lbs. She had a complete oral rehabilitation as part of her many surgeries. Before she lost her weight, she had been so heavy that she simply would not fit in a dental chair even if one could be found capable of handling that much weight. As a result, she was not able to visit a dentist for many years. Because of this forced neglect, several of her teeth had to be removed, and she also needed many root canals and crowns. Her dentistry was reported to have been done in 7 all-day appointments over a 3 week period. Now that's an aggressive timeline.

The show pays

In other shows you see people that have crowns, caps, placed on their misshapen or misaligned front and back teeth. The miracle of such shows is that within several weeks the patients are completely made over: ears fixed, noses realigned, liposuctions performed, skin rejuvenated and tightened, and a brand new smile that would make most Hollywood stars envious. The good news for these patients is that "The Show" managed to get the dentistry done at no fee for the patient. Either the show paid for the work, or the dentist did not charge and performed the work for the exposure they received by making these folks beautiful.

I have often wondered if the dentists made it clear to the patients that this work has a definite life expectancy. It will have to be redone at some point, possibly more than once. The only question is how long before the makeover will have to be made over?

A whole new area of dentistry

These very cases that seem so wonderful when seen on TV have spawned a whole new industry, aesthetic dentistry. Some feel it should be a specialty. In fact, there is recognized specialty of Prosthetic Dentistry that qualifies dentists to do such complex restorative work. To be board certified in this specialty takes 3 to 4 years of work beyond dental school. These boarded dentists are very well trained in these types of cases. From my years of experience I am more than happy to send such cases to a specialist. The problems begin when such cases are attempted by dentists who are not so thoroughly trained.

Cosmetic, aesthetic, dentistry

The cosmetic dentistry cases vary from very simple cases of bleaching, which any dentist can to do, through porcelain veneers in order to slightly change the shape of teeth. Then the cases become more complex, ranging from missing and poorly positoned teeth that require veneers, crowns, bridges, orthodontics and, in the worst cases orthognathic surgery, jaw surgery, to realign the jaws. Before we look at some of your options, let's first determine when you should consider the procedure.

When is cosmetic dentistry right for you?

We have all seen these shows where an average-looking person undergoes some magic and comes out looking like a movie star. And most of us have probably wondered what it would be like to have that perfect smile, perfect figure, perfect look. It seems within reach to achieve this, if only we were willing and able to spend a little bit of money and suffer a little bit of pain.

Success does not hinge on having a perfect smile. Look at some of our most successful people. David Letterman has a large gap between his front teeth, but David is a master of the interview and a fast retort. Condoleezza Rice has gaps between her front teeth large enough to harbor weapons of mass destruction. Being Secretary of State as a black woman with a large gap certainly makes you wonder what Rice might have achieved had her smile been perfect. Jay Leno has a lower jaw that is 5 sizes too large, but his comedy timing is precise. What did all these people have in common? They were very successful.

You too can have it all

The aesthetic dentists' ads paint an enticing picture. You come in and have your teeth done, and everything will suddenly fall into place. Your life will be different. You will be more successful. You will find a better job and make more money. You will have more fun. Your sex life will be wonderful. You no longer will frighten your grandchildren when you smile. Just come and sit in the dentist chair and it will all be taken care of for you. But when you think about it, can it really be that simple?

It's true that a beautiful smile will give you confidence, and you will look in the mirror with pleasure. If that's what you are after, and if you fully understand the limitations of each treatment, by all means, go for it. But no dentist, no matter how skilled, can do more than improve your smile. The treatment won't change the heart of an unfaithful spouse, nor will it make your children behave any better. It won't even shorten your commute. So think realistically what you can expect of your dental work before you take the plunge.

There have been studies where a patient's self esteem was measured before and after cosmetic surgery. Immediately after the surgery they did show an increase in self esteem. However, within a short time, in just a few months they were right back where they started.

This chapter will help you decide which treatment, if any, is right for you. It will also help you avoid pitfalls set up by some less than scrupulous dentists. Finally, you will learn how to choose the dentist you can trust to do a good job for you at a fair price.

Remember, nothing the best dentist does will be as good as what Mother Nature gave you. Natural teeth that have not decayed or chipped are much stronger, and will last longer than any veneer, crown, bridge, or implant. Keep this in mind when you are making your decision about an elective dental procedure.

Bleaching

Americans believe the correct color of teeth is that of a Chicklet. Just look at popular actors, TV personalities, or models on covers of magazines. Every one of them has teeth so pearly white that if they got any whiter we would need sunglasses! If your teeth are not the color of new fallen snow, you must try harder.

Carbamide peroxide, or Glyoxide, is a chemical we have used for more than the last 40 years. It is a form of hydrogen peroxide that helped clean out infected areas around the teeth and gums. I had used this for years but never noticed the adjacent teeth got whiter. Someone did and we were off to the brightness wars.

You can bleach your teeth very inexpensively.

For many years I had patients make their own bite guard bleaching trays and I gave them a bottle of Glyoxide. No cost, just a way for me to say thank you for coming to me. If they used it every night, their teeth would be noticeably whiter in two weeks. Other dentists went from the 5% carbamide peroxide in Glyoxide to 10%, 25%, even 30% and the teeth got much whiter faster. They also tended to get very sensitive to hot and cold. You can also use whitening strips. While they cost a little more, they are still inexpensive and very convenient.

Laser bleaching

You can go more hi-tech with your bleaching. Companies came out with laser bleaching; remember, if it is laser it must be good. You went in and they painted the teeth with the 30% and aimed a "laser" that turned out to be a bright light and in an hour you left with a dazzling smile, and a very sensitive set of teeth. Interestingly, one of the research organizations was testing the light system when the light went out. They called the company and asked what to do since they were half way through the bleaching. They were told the chemical works just as well without the light. Some dentists are charging $700 for this instantaneous whitening, others even more. Those lasers really work. The company that has the machines will place them in your office for part of the fee. Of course you are obligated to use it a minimum number of times a month. Do you suppose that tends to increase the chance that you need bleaching?

Bleaching works and it has been done long enough we are comfortable that it is safe. But some people take it to extremes. Patients have been reported to have bleached so much that they have lost most of the color in their teeth. The teeth start to look grey because they are translucent. Too much of a good thing is a bad thing.

About 40 years ago I had a patient come into the office for an emergency. She had a toothache. However, she had the whitest teeth I had ever seen. They were toilet bowl, snow, bright white. This was long before veneers or bleaching.

As I started to examine her I also noticed some of her gum tissue was white. I was at a bit of a loss. White patches on the gum tissue can be a precursor of cancer, and certainly an indicator of irritation. The first step is to see if it wipes off. I took a gauze square and the white wiped off leaving a normal gum tissue. That was a good sign. However I also had managed to wipe some of the white off her teeth.

I asked her if she knew what the white coating was from. She said, "I want white teeth. I brush 4 times a day. I used brightening toothpaste. I even tried a smoker's toothpaste and I do not smoke. Nothing seems to work. (Remember this was prior to bleaching.) So I got some white fingernail polish and I paint my teeth white.

Unfortunately her hand eye coordination was not real good and it is very hard to paint your own teeth working in a mirror. So she would also get some

*of the white polish on her gums. It did no damage
and I had to appreciate her inventiveness. Today
of course, she probably would have Chiclets with
the advent of bleaching systems.*

Changing the shape of your teeth

What if you have crooked, crowded teeth,
or if you have unsightly spaces between your
teeth, or teeth that will not bleach as white as
you wish? For the misaligned teeth the best
solution is orthodontic treatment, or braces.
Braces can be used by both adults and kids.
Adults take a little longer. However, in the world
of instant communication, instant gratification,
liposuction, thermage, etc., we in dentistry
simply have to do better than that, and we have.
It is called the instant makeover, smile design, or
aesthetic dentistry. Dental professionals doing
this work have an organization, the American
Association of Cosmetic Dentistry. This tends to
indicate the rest of us are unaesthetic dentists.

Veneers

Veneers are the fake fingernail of dentistry.
They can be made of acrylic, composites, or
porcelain. They are thin shells that fit over the
existing teeth making them a brighter color,
closing spaces, or changing the shape to give
a more regular arrangement. They can mask
badly stained teeth. Such changes require very
little reduction of the tooth's enamel, which is a
good thing—remember, we cannot grow new
enamel. When it is flushed down the suction it is
gone for ever. The less that is removed, the less

trauma the nerve of the tooth has to go through. It is rare for one of these teeth to require a root canal because of this trauma from this minor reduction, and therefore you will have more options in the future.

Well done veneers can serve you well, but if they are not done right, you can have some nasty surprises. I once went on a cruise. One of the folks there was the father-in-law of a dentist, and his son was also a dentist. The father's veneer came off on the trip. He was going to visit my home town after the cruise, so I volunteered to re-cement the veneer. When I got the father in the office and took a look at the now veneerless tooth, the sucking sound you could hear was my breath. I expected a bit of enamel removed and a healthy tooth now exposed. To my shock, there was less than 1/4th of the tooth left. It would have been much more conservative to have gone to a full crown. I re-cemented the veneer and thanked the dental god that the father lived in some other part of the country, because I knew this was not going to work. I found out later that the veneer had come off again less than a week later. I have no idea what the son-in-law was going to do, but I was relieved I was not the one having to face the situation of a veneer that had been badly over-prepared in the quest for the perfect smile. I hoped the quest had been initiated by the father-in-law, but I feared it had been the dentist's idea. After all, the man was in his 70's and was a little overweight, balding, had some skin defects, and clearly showed his age. Did the teeth really make enough difference to justify this sort of treatment?

How much will beauty cost?

What sort of costs are we looking at for veneers?

First we need to address how many veneers you want. If you just want a beautiful smile, you can limit yourself to 6, 8, or maybe 10 upper teeth. Now, if you want to be beautiful when you grimace and smile, you need both upper and lower arches, so we are up to 12 to 20 teeth, including the anterior and bicuspids of each arch. I have seen composites done for under $400 a tooth, a mere $8,000 total. Now, if you want the most beautiful porcelain, it will cost about $950 a tooth, for a total of just under $20,000. And if you go to a spa office with a member of the AACD, particularly if they do some presentations for the AACD, plan on $2000 a tooth or more. These self proclaimed experts might very well tap your retirement fund for $40,000.

How long will they last?

How long will veneers last? That is a bit hard to predict. I have seen numerous requests for redoes while doing insurance reviews of composite (plastic) veneers less than 5 years old. How does this happen? Some will break. They simply are not as strong as teeth. The composite veneer depends on having a strong tooth underneath. It's very much like a fake fingernail, only covering the front surface of a tooth. This can be very acceptable is some cases, but don't expect them to last for the rest of your life. In 7- 10 years colors will change or they will stain. In a very clean mouth 10 years is probably close to the maximum life expectancy of these veneers.

All-porcelain veneers are quite strong and will likely last longer. For teeth that are out of position it might be necessary to remove up to half of the structure above the gum tissue. The longevity of these depends on a strong bond to the remaining tooth for strength. Sometimes this bond is just not that strong or the patient puts much more stress on the veneer than it can withstand. I had one patient who broke her veneers 3 times. I finally had to go to a crown to get strength.

The gums will recede

Over time, some veneers will develop stains where the veneer ends and the tooth begins at the gum line. This can be due to a bad bond, a gap due to bad fit, or simply recession of the gum tissue that exposes dark root surface. Some patients will develop decay, probably because the veneers did not fit well. Some dentists have told me that their veneers last 15 years. It is possible but there is no guarantee. And even these "long lasting veneers" will need to be replaced, possibly multiple times if the patient is young.

> *I recently received a magazine with an article from one of the experts who runs an institute. He showed a young woman with a beautiful smile who was running in a state beauty contest. Her smile was not perfect, however, so he did veneers. She now had a spectacular smile. Seven years later she had just turned 30 and her gum tissue had receded enough to show some roots. His solution was to do a new set of veneers. She shows*

a lot of teeth when she smiles. You can do the calculations as to how many sets of veneers she will go through in a lifetime. It is harder to figure out when the veneers will have to be crowns and how many crowns will need to be redone or how many will need root canals.

Crowns

A more drastic solution than veneers is crowns, or caps. To put a crown in, your dentist must remove all of the enamel and replace it with either an all porcelain crown or metal and porcelain one. The difference is strength. The metal and porcelain crown is 50% stronger than natural tooth and all porcelain that is about 80% as strong as natural tooth. The all-porcelain crown has better color and translucency, thus looking more natural. However, you need to be in good light and be using magnification for the average non-dentist to tell the difference. The all porcelain crown requires removal of more tooth structure. This probably leads to more nerves dying. If the nerve dies you will need a root canal. Because your root is now not easily accessible, a hole must be drilled through the all porcelain crown, weakening it. Sometimes the porcelain crown will break. In general, the current best guess is that 1 nerve in 10 will die after a crown and require a root canal. The metal and porcelain crowns require a bit less reduction and maybe only 1 nerve in 20 will die. The more structure that is removed the greater the stress on the dental nerve and the greater the chance that it will die. If the nerve dies, you can make a hole in the metal portion without significantly weakening the crown. Fortunately, fixing this problem is a simple matter of placing a filling in the hole that was drilled to access the nerve chamber. I have done this successfully for 40 years. Some dentists will insist on redoing the crown if a root canal access has been made, but in my experience it is not usually necessary.

An even more drastic solution is to remove the teeth and place implants with crowns. Cost can be over $4,000 per tooth and implant. It can take more than a year from start to finish. It is much more traumatic. We will talk about implants later in this chapter.

Why not crown them all

So long as we are crowning teeth, why not simply crown all 14 uppers and 14 lowers? The cost is $950 to $2000 a tooth. You do the math; I get dizzy when considering such numbers. Add in 3 or 4 root canals if you are lucky and only have that many teeth die after the trauma of all these crown preps. You just made the dentist's week. It is time for a new Porsche. Now if you get lucky and find a truly great dentist, you will end up with a beautiful smile. You will look natural from ear to ear. When you go into acting and your face appears on the big screen and you scream showing all your teeth, no one will know you ever had an amalgam filling. Your smile will truly be spectacular. That is the good news. The bad news is that it is difficult, if not impossible, to pick such a dentist. And if you want to choose based on their marketing alone, I have a bridge in Brooklyn I would like to talk to you about. I can get you a fair price for the bridge. Remember in 15 to 20 years it will have to be redone.

Some unscrupulous dentists will do the work on patients even when it goes clearly against the patient's best interest. Let's look a real life scenario I have encountered: a 70 year old man whose bridge broke. It affected 4 teeth, and the bridge needed to be redone. The man went to a dentist who advertised himself as an aesthetic expert. The dentist properly diagnosed decay, and informed the patient that the bridge needed to be redone. It was a 4 tooth bridge that would cost in the $3,000 to $4,000 range in the average office in 2004.

But, unknown to the patient, the dentist had attended a weekend seminar to the institute we described above, and was about to attend another. He explained to the patient how with his aesthetic expertise he could give him the smile of a Dallas Cowboys cheerleader. He neglected to remind his patient that most of the cheer leaders are in their 20s and he was in his 70s.

He neglected to appreciate that the patient was over 70 years old, had heart problems that required him to take a number of medications, including nitroglycerine, on an almost daily basis. This indicates that he had rather severe heart disease and needed to avoid stress. The dentist was so "helpful" that he gave the patient a special deal: the patient could come to the institute in the Southwest and he would give him a special price for the dentistry.

See the problem? The dentist could not call himself a specialist, as there was no specialty of aesthetic dentistry. The average patient does not recognize this subtle nuance. The dentist convinced the patient that all his teeth needed to be crowned and he wanted to use this patient at one of these institutes. He would fly him to the big city, put him up in a hotel and give him a 50% discount in fees. It all sounded very alluring, a deal of a lifetime. On top of the great financial deal, the patient would have the smile he always wanted, he would not scare his grandchildren when he smiled. Making friends would be easier. His life would now be different. The teeth were all prepped; many required root canals.

It turned out the patient had had bypass surgery 2 years earlier and still had major cardiac problems that required daily medication to control pain of angina.

Unaware of the danger, the patient agreed and went to the big city and the dentist started cutting down his teeth for crowns—not just the 4 involved in the bridge but all his upper teeth. Some of the teeth needed root canals before he was done cutting them down for crowns. These were done as the day went on. By 3 in the afternoon the patient was exhausted and was taking heart medicine to control chest pain. At this point the dentist decided to stop. This was possibly the only wise decision he had made that day. In fact, it probably saved the patient's life. He had given him 22 cartridges of local anesthesia. Nine is considered to be the maximum safe dose. Because the anesthesia was given over 8 hours, the patient luckily survived.

But the ordeal was not over. The patient went to the hotel to rest and recover after the exhausting day in the dental chair. He looked in the mirror and got suspicious about the quality of the temporaries. He now sought a second opinion. This independent dentist was much less complimentary than the institute instructors. The patient was sent for a second opinion of the root canals and yet a third and 4th opinion. All came out badly.

At this point, the patient's wife went in and argued with the treating dentist about the work that had been done. The session was very stressful, and eventually the wife was told to leave the office. She had a heart attack that night and died. The dentist was brought up on a complaint of bad temporaries. He beat these accusations; no one looked at the bad patient selection. No one looked at the overdose of local anesthesia that could have killed the patient. The patient needed a simple 4 tooth bridge, was elderly, had a bad heart and ended up with a bunch of root canals and crowns on all his teeth. After the 4th opinion, it was decided that things were so bad the only solution was to take out all the man's teeth and go to dentures. After he healed they could place some implants to stabilize the dentures. God only knows how much more money crossed the table.

Some time later as an instructor in dental sedation I got a call from the first dentist. He said, "I think if I could have done oral sedation I could have finished the case."

I said, "No, you cannot come to my course. It is full already."

But the dentist was persistent. "When will you have another class?" he asked

"I said no, don't come to my class. You do not

have common sense, and I cannot teach you that in a weekend course. In his case I probably could not have done it in a two year course."

How long will crowns last?

I have many patients with crowns that are over 25 years old, some even over 35 years old. With time, the gum tissue will recede, exposing root. If the roots are kept clean the crowns can last for a long time. As we get older it gets harder to do a good job of cleaning. Using a daily fluoride gel can help. Fluoride varnish applied in the dental office can help as well.

You must brush teeth with crowns

I have seen people get decay on an exposed root in as little as 5 years. Why would this be? One cause is that some people only brush their teeth on Sundays of leap years. If you decide to have crowns, it is absolutely vital that you brush regularly.

I have seen insurance submissions for crown remakes in as little as 3 years. This usually suggests the crown did not fit well, and there was a gap between the tooth and the crown that food and bacteria got into.

Porcelain crowns can break. This can happen if you hit a rock, a piece of bone, if you chew ice or fingernails or if you clench your teeth. It is one of the risks of porcelain crowns particularly all-porcelain, non metallic crowns.

The gums will recede

One further problem is the slow recession of the gum tissue. When the crowns are placed, the margin where the crown joins the tooth is under the gum and everything is wonderful. A few years later the gums have receded and the metal margin of the crown shows, or the dark root surface is exposed. If that bothers you, the solution is a new crown.

Crowns are an insult to the nerve of the tooth

Each time a crown is redone, it is an insult to the nerve and increases the risk of the tooth needing a root canal. It has been estimated that if a simple filling is needed in a back tooth, that will cause, on the average, an expenditure of $2,100 in 2001 dollars over a lifetime of a patient. Some patients might go 5 or 10 times this. One filling will lead to a larger filling and that to a larger filling, eventually requiring a crown that will need to be replaced some day, and possibly the nerve will die at some point and the tooth will require a root canal. This scenario is particularly true if you switch dentists often. With modest inflation that figure can double or triple.

Implants

To simplify our discussion, I will describe the process of placing an implant. First, you must have adequate amounts of bone to place the implant. If a tooth has been removed, you will probably have to wait until the bone has filled in the hole where the root was. If there is inadequate bone, grafts of artificial bone or freeze dried bone might be necessary. Once the bone is adequate, the overlying tissue is laid open and a hole the same size and shape as the implant is drilled into the bone. The implant will be selected that will fit the hole in the bone. The implants are made of titanium, or similar non-reactive metal that is inert to the body. The body does not react to the material so it is not rejected. In many ways the implant is the size and shape of a bolt with no head. The implant is threaded, screwed, into the bone. The gum tissue is then sutured over the implant and the jaw is allowed to heal for 6 to 9 months. After healing, a minor surgery is done to uncover the top of the implant and a post is screwed into the implant. This post comes through the gum tissue and serves as a tooth that a crown, bridge, or denture can be attached to.

There is a new trend to place implants at the time a tooth is extracted and to place the crown on the implant immediately. Only time will show if this works.

Implants last

The best evidence as of 2006 is that implants work and appear to be as long lasting, and possibly even longer lasting than bridge work that has been used for years to replace missing teeth. We have come a long way. Implants that were done 30 years ago only lasted 10 – 15 years. The implants being done today may have double the 10 to 15 year life expectancy. It is too soon to know because such implants have only been around about 20 years. But they are looking good at this point. Uppers probably do not hold up quite as well because the upper bone is spongier.

Implants are costly

The bad news is, implants are costly. In 2006 it was not uncommon to see one implant cost $3000 or perhaps more if bone grafting was necessary. It is possible to place 10 implants, crown these implants adding fake teeth where no implant has been placed as you would do for a bridge, and in this way replace a denture with a bridge that replaces all the missing teeth in an upper or lower arch. You can do the math, this can cost over $60,000, or more, if you are getting rid of upper and lower dentures. But it is as close to natural teeth as possible if you have lost all your teeth.

There are several other uses of implants and many different types of implants. One recent development has to do with orthodontics. To move teeth, you need anchor teeth to serve as a base for the braces to apply a force to move anterior, or front, teeth. If you are an adult and have lost your back teeth, an implant can be placed to serve as that anchor.

Mini implants

In the early 2000s, a mini implant came to market. It looks like a small wood screw made of titanium about 1.8 mm, 1/32 of an inch, in diameter, with a small ball on the top. The ball looks like a mini trailer hitch. These have been a godsend for denture wearers.

Find that super dentist

Let's see how we might go about our search for this gifted dentist. What if the dentist claims to be a graduate of one of the institutes, and further claims to be one of the top dentists in the world because of his or her training? If you look, you will see many ads stating this or that dentist is one of the top 5% of dentists in the country. This dentist was voted as one of the best dentists in the US by his or her peers. This sounds impressive, so let's take a closer look. The problem is, anyone who pays tuition can go to such an institution. No one flunks out; everyone gets in and everyone graduates. The only selection criterion is the ability to beg, borrow, or buy your way into a weekend class. There is no mechanism to determine who the best dentist in the country is. There is no voting as to who is the best. At least I have never been sent a ballot and I have been around a long time. Clearly, this is not the best way to pick the right dentist to do your crowns.

The institutes

There are regional dental institutes that are usually not associated with a dental school. They all have web pages. These web pages tell all about the advantages to a dentist who had taken one of their courses. Their courses run from $2000 to $8,000 for the dentist. Even so, they state on their web site: *"However, even though doctors have been through our programs, we can't assure the public that they absorbed the knowledge we presented, or grasp the important concepts of aesthetic restorative neuromuscular dentistry."* This sounds to me like a copout.

Several are attempting to start a Mastership program. This is a self-proclaimed competency that is available to those who take enough courses and are willing to purchase the wall plaque. I am somewhat suspicious when the award is made by the same organization that sells the course you must take in order to qualify for the award, and determines if your credentials are adequate.

I have seen ads stating that these institute graduates are the top 5% of dentists in the country. It just so happens that about 5% of the dentists in the country have taken one of their courses. I know of no certifying, independent body that attempts to rank dentists.

Cosmetic dentistry = money

Cosmetic dentistry has become a very lucrative business. All dentists are cosmetic, aesthetic dentists. No dentist would be categorized as a non-aesthetic dentist. Depending on the severity of the aesthetic problem, you might need someone with special training. Only those with Dental School advanced degrees, MSD, assure you of the quality of advanced training a dentist might have. Beyond going to such a specialist, all other designations are of lesser importance. Do you need an MSD? Probably not, unless you have special, severe problems. In any case, shop around, ask questions, look at the dentist's photo albums (be sure they are photos of the dentist's work—remember the dentist can buy such photos) and not their brochures, ask more questions, talk to satisfied patients and above all, be critical of any claims that are made.

> *Some dentists advertise on TV, in the weekly newspaper supplements, in the phone book, in supermarket slick brochures, mailing, and radio, on billboards and on the side of buses. Guess who pays for the advertising?*

Do not assume that the photos in a dentist's brochure or hanging on their office walls illustrate that dentist's work. These images are available for sale by various vendors. The only valid credential that you can be sure are indicative of advanced skill is a Masters degree in restorative dentistry from a US dental school. You will find people with this credential in the Yellow Pages under prosthodontist. This is a specialty of dentistry, and you will find behind their names the letters DDS MSD or DMD MSD. If you don't see these initials, the dentist probably has not taken specialty training.

What other letters you might see in the Yellow Pages mean

What does PS mean behind the dentist's name? It simply means they are a corporation, and it is not an advanced degree. You might see FAGD, FASDA, FACAD, FICI, FALD. LVI, AACD, ICI, ALD. These are simply organizations the dentist belongs to. They do not necessarily imply or guarantee any special knowledge.

Many folks who practice and advertise "aesthetic dentistry," "the miracle smile makeover," "smile design," "dazzling smile," "cosmetic and laser dentistry," "advanced tooth whitening," "sleep dentistry," are masters at marketing but might not have the skills to match their ads. Many are really good at doing a financial procedure known as a wallet biopsy.

It is OK to have the smile you always wanted

There are some good reasons to do aesthetic makeovers. If you wake up every morning, smile in the mirror and hate yourself and your smile, that is a good reason to do something. If you have multiple missing teeth, have to wear partial dentures and would like teeth that were much like your original teeth in that they were not loose and did not have to be removed to clean, implants and bridges can come close to giving you back what you once had. The importance of this book and this chapter is that it is your choice. Do not let Dr. Do Lots of Make

Overs sell you dentistry you do not need and do not want.

Age relevant dentistry

There is a concept known as age relevant dentistry. At the age of 55 it may make sense to do a lot of crowns. They may need to be redone at 65 to 75 but probably will not be an issue when you are 90. At 90 your priorities will be different. Medically you might not be up to another make over and you probably will not expect to look like you are 30. However, if you start the process at 20 years of age, it may not be possible to redo the makeover the number of times that will be required by the time you are 90. What does not make sense at 20 may be a rational decision at 55 or 60. Realize that once this process is started it will have to be redone every few years. Do not let a fast talker schmooze you into work that you do not want and that is not necessary.

Buyer Beware.

14. Periodontics

Your teeth are great, but the gum's got to go.

Periodontic, perio, refers to the tissue surrounding the teeth.

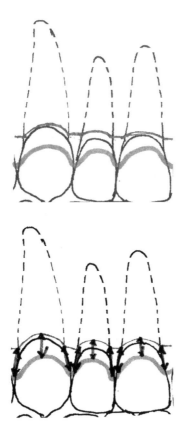

Figure 14.1 A healthy mouth has high gum and high levels of bone. If we measure the distance from the gum level to the bone level, we will find pocket up to 3 mm in a healthy mouth.

A healthy mouth has high gum and high levels of bone

If we measure the distance from the gum level to the bone level, we will find pockets up to 3 mm. in a healthy mouth.

Step one - Gingivitis

When I graduated from dental school it was very simple. If you left food and bacteria around your teeth the gingival (gum) tissue would become inflamed and red, and would bleed easily because the inflammation or redness happened because of additional blood vessels and vessels that were dilated. If you touched the tissues, blood leaked from the tissue. This was referred to as gingivitis, inflammation of the gingival.

Step two - Periodontitis

If you did not get serious about cleaning, this gingivitis would spread to the underlying tissues disrupting the connective tissue. This was periodontitis. If you continued to ignore the problem the bone around and between the teeth would be resorbed and eventually lost.

Step three - Pocket formation

This led to pocket formation. We use a fine probe and slide it between the tooth and the gum tissue. As this advances, it will eventually stop at the level where the gingival tissue attaches to the tooth. It is believed that this attachment is a little more than one mm. from the bone level. By measuring the distance of the periodontal pocket, we can get an indication of where the bone is.

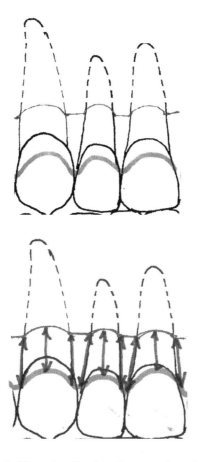

Figure 14.2 The teeth in these drawings have advanced bone loss. The tissue is many millimeters above where the tissue actually attaches to the teeth. A third to half of the original bone has been lost.

I just condensed several years of studies into 3 paragraphs. When I graduated from dental school it was very simple. You cleaned the plaque, food, and bacteria, and calculus (hard deposits) off the teeth both above and below the tissue level and the tissue returned to health and the problem was solved.

Pockets

If the patient ignored the bleading tissue, bone was lost and pockets developed. The pockets made it more difficult for the patient and dentist to clean these teeth because the spaces below the level of the gum tissue could not be reached by a brush and, if the pockets were more than 6 mm. it was difficult if not impossible for the dentist or dental hygienist to do a perfect job of cleaning. In addition these cleanings known as root planing scaling are painful often requiring local anesthesia.

Eliminate pockets

The solution was to mow the grass, cut off the extra tissue above the bone. This was referred to as a gingivectomy, a circumcism of the gums. This left the teeth longer with root exposure but in theory they were easier for the patient and the dentist to clean. If they were kept clean the bone would not be lost.

The pockets are back so I went to school

The problem was, 10 years later we again had pockets. I was failing my patients. So I joined a periodontal study club. I spent one day a month for 3 years with experts from the dental school learning new techniques.

I used these techniques for the next 10 years and people kept getting worse. I decided I just could not do this work so I sent patients to the specialists who had taught the study club. Ten years later the patients I had referred were still loosing bone.

The new concept of perio disease

I should emphasize that we all lose bone as we age. If we are lucky (more about this later) and are good home care artists, the bone loss should be very slow. I have patients in their 80s who look as good as 30 year olds (that is the level of their bone). In the late 1990s, I attended a symposium that was a paradigm shift.

Perio is a genetic disease

Experts from all over the world discussed periodontal problems. I came away knowing refractory periodontal disease, that disease that seemed to progress regardless of what patients and their dentists did, was a genetic disease. Inflammation in these patients was controlled by several genes. If you got the two bad genes you would lose bone and probably teeth at an early age. If you smoked, you would lose them even earlier. You could slow the progression some if you were a super star in home care and got your teeth cleaned every two or three months. However, the outcome was determined more by your genes than your home care and what your dentist could do.

Surgery may not be the best option

The surgery we had been taught probably did not influence the outcome much if at all. The one factor that we could change was smoking. One very prominent specialist stated that if we wanted to make a difference we should have smoking cessation programs as that was the one thing we could do that works.

This was very bad news for periodontists, those specialists who treated gum disease. Most of what they had been doing did not have good long-term effect.

At about the same time, implants became popular. The periodontist had good surgical technique and started doing implants. I much prefer implants placed by periodontists as they generally are more gentle to the tissues and they better understand the problems I would have as a restorative dentist if I did not get the implants properly aligned.

Perio, heart disease, and preterm deliveries

The symposium presented other findings. The genes that controlled inflammation also seemed to have an effect on coronary artery disease and low birth weight babies (premature births). The inflammatory effect seemed to lead to plaque formations in vessels and cause premature labor.

Note I did not state that periodontal problems caused heart problems or premature deliveries. All three were caused by this gene defect. One is a marker for the other but there is no cause and effect.

For the last 7 or 8 years there have been many attempts to prove that coronary vessel plaque, even strokes and premature deliveries, are all caused by periodontal disease. If this is ever proven we will all beat a path to the door of dentists to get our teeth cleaned. We will do this to keep from dying of heart disease or stroke but we will not always do it to save our teeth. As of today, there has yet to be a study that shows cause and effect. There certainly is a relationship. Both are caused by the gene defect.

C reactive protein, CRP

Recently we are seeing a new player, C reactive Protein, CRP. CRP is produced by the liver and is only present during episodes of acute inflammation. There is a test for CRP that gives a general indication of acute inflammation. This can check for a number of inflammatory diseases, rheumatoid arthritis, and lupus. It is not 100% predictive.

Recently there have been studies that show CRP is elevated in heart attacks. It has not been ascertained if it is an indication of the damage or if it plays a role in causing the atherosclerotic disease. Some researchers are making the claim that elevated levels of CRP may cause the problem. They are quick to point out the periodontal disease may contribute to the elevated levels of CRP. Some dentists who believe this are selling nutritional supplements to help decrease the level of CRP, decreasing the thickness of plaque deposits in the coronary arteries and, of course, in the process thicken their wallets .

Maybe some day we will be able to say we can prevent heart attacks, strokes, and premature deliveries, but as of 2007 there is no evidence that periodontal disease causes these other problems. The truth as we now know it is the cells that line our blood vessels can produce CRP. This CRP helps produce plaque that can block these vessels and can cause clots. One of the ways to reduce this is with Statin drugs, Zocor and Crestor. Treating other risk factors such as smoking, obesity, high blood pressure, and high cholesterol all lower CRP. It is a big leap of faith to believe that treating periodontal disease will have the same effect. Taking nutritional supplements is even a bigger leap.

15. Endodontics – root canals

Am I paying for a root canal or the Panama Canal

In concept, doing a root canal is quite simple. The devil is in the details. In practice they can be maddeningly difficult.

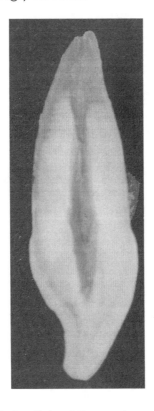

Figure 15.1 This tooth had 1 canal
The pulp, nerve, is found in the chamber in the middle of the tooth and its root. In this tooth the

hole at the apex of the root can be seen. Blood vessels and nerve tissue pass through the hole.

Diagnosis

First we need a diagnosis. The reason for root canal is usually a dying, dead, or infected nerve in a tooth. The classic symptoms is pain, one of the most intense pains known to man. Often cooling the tooth can control this pain. The difficult diagnosis is when a nerve is dying. The tooth may be sensitive to hot or cold or both. It may be sensitive to bite. The pain may come and go. I just described almost every toothache I have ever seen. Only a small part of them needed endo.

In general, if it kept you awake last night, if the pain can be stopped by cold water or, if there is swelling, your nerve has died. We think that, at the first signs of pain, the connective tissue starts to swell in the pulp chamber. This increase in pressure shuts off the blood supply to the pulp. This causes the tissue to die as it is not getting nutrients and oxygen. Unfortunately, the nerve tissue is still alive because the cell body of the nerve cell is in the cranial cavity. Only an extension of this nerve is in the tooth.

Cold may help the pain

The nerve tissue becomes overly sensitive because of the irritation of the dying pulp tissue. As this tissue dies it will often cause gas to form. The gas can be under high pressure.

This stimulates the nerve tissue further. Cold will shrink the gas, decreasing the pressure. This is why ice water often helps the pain and is diagnostic of a dead nerve.

Swelling and infection is the next problem

Eventually all the tissue in the tooth dies and it leaks out the tip of the root causing an infection of the bone tissue at the tips of the root. This causes pressure, more pain, and elevates the tooth in its socket. Now every time you close your teeth you hit the tooth driving it into this area of infection causing more pain and trauma. Eventually, the infection erodes through the bone causing the soft tissues of your face to swell. When this happens, the pain often gets better because the pressure in the bone releases. You now have an infection that can lead to a systemic life threatening crisis.

Altitude

Some patients will notice pain when flying. The average commercial jet is pressurized at 5 to 9 thousand feet, which is less than the pressure at sea level. The gas pressure differential will be greater at altitude. There was a time in WWII when all aircrews had their fillings replaced because of fear that gas was captured under the fillings. These crews flew above 20,000 feet, with the aid of oxygen. Many of this pain probably was associated with nerves that were dying. Similarly, diving causes an increase pressure that can trigger tooth pain. If either of these happen get to a dentist.

The moral: get to the dentist if you are having pain.

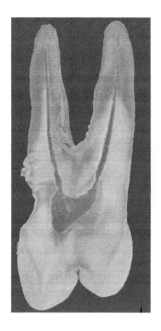

Figure 15.2 This is a tooth with 2 canals.

Open the chamber

Our first step after we have determined that a nerve is dying is to get pain control. This can be very difficult in the early stages because you have an alive, inflamed, traumatized nerve in a pool of dying tissue. It can be a challenge to get numbness under these circumstances. However, if we do not proceed, the pain will increase very dramatically over the next day. In the later stages, when the chamber is full of puss (infection), that portion of the nerve in the pulp chamber may be dead, and no local anesthesia is necessary.

Next, we must open into the pulp chamber. As our bur opens this chamber, we may see gas or puss escape. We have released the pressure that has been causing the pain.

I went to the office one morning at 3 AM to see a patient in extreme pain. He met me with cup of ice water. My diagnosis was made. I only had to determine which was the offending tooth. Again all he had to do was to touch the tooth and he would pale. With step number two done, I opened the pulp chamber and had puss squirt 5 feet. He then went to sleep. I shook him to wake him up. He said, "this is wonderful. I have not slept in 3 days." I had to perk a pot of coffee to get him awake enough to leave the office.

At this point, we can leave the tooth open to drain and plan an appointment to finish the endo. Some would argue that the tooth should be sealed up with medication. The problem I have seen with this is the fact that often the tooth will build pressure and I will be back in the office during off hours. This is a point to be argued by dentists. I leave them open, while others insist they must be sealed.

This tooth gives you an idea of just how small the pulp chamber can be as it goes down the root. This tooth has what would be considered a rather large chamber. Many are finer than a thin thread

Clean out the dying tissue

Now is a time to clean out all the dead and dying tissue. We use a series of graded files to do this. The problem is that the pulp and pulp chamber is not an even taper, nor is it round and it often has accessory canals that go out the side of the root and when we get to the tip of the root there may be a plexus of paths rather than one. All of this leads to stress for the dentist. It is important to get rid of all the pulp tissue. It is also almost impossible to do this with just files. For this reason, we will irrigate the canal with a Clorox mixture to dissolve any tissue we cannot get to.

Seal the canal

Next, we dry the canal with very small paper points, introduce some cement into the canal and finally seal the chamber. The standard had been Gutta percha although we are beginning to see some plastics. With a perfect seal, the tooth becomes comfortable, the swelling goes down, sometimes with the aid of an antibiotic.

Back teeth with endo will need crowns

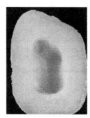

Figure 15.3 This molar has three canals this is looking down into the canals from the top of the tooth.

Most posterior endo teeth will need a crown, although I have placed silver amalgam fillings in many of them when a patient could not afford a crown and have had many go for years. The process of gaining access into posterior teeth removes a major part of the top of the tooth that will weaken it some. I really think all molars and most bicuspids should be crowned. Front (anterior) teeth do not routinely need crowns if there is no other breakdown.

Some dentists will routinely place metal posts into one or more of the canals and charge for a build up. This is only necessary if the tooth was so badly broken down that you cannot get a 3 mm band (ferrule) of solid tooth when the crown is prepared. If this ferrule is not possible, there are those who believe the crown prep should be taken further down the tooth. The posts that are placed for buildups are last ditch attempts to get retention to hold a crown. These posts should not routinely be placed in front teeth as they weaken the root.

I had a tooth get sensitive on a Monday but I was busy. On Tuesday it was worse, but my associate dentist had a busy schedule and I did not want to bother her. Wednesday I practiced alone. I was getting more and more pain but I am tough. I am Swedish. Thursday was a very busy day for both of us and the pain was better. Friday I went hiking in the mountains chasing the Japanese pine mushroom that grows under fir trees (another story). It was a marvelous day. I got more 'rooms that day than I had in some years. I also got hammered by my tooth every time I bent over.

I got home in time to go to the office but I was dirty and had 'rooms to clean. Saturday was not a good day. But I could not disrupt this very busy day for my associate. After all, I could have come in all week. By Sunday I could walk on water. But I really could not have her come in on her day off because of my stupidity. I was in the office bright and early on Monday. She opened the tooth and the relief was wonderful. I had the endo done and 2 years later I still get a twinge of pain every now and again.

We think what happens is that when we have a tooth die and experience severe pain for several days we teach the nerve to send pain signals. Much as we learn other things we can learn pain. This is also known as "phantom pain." People who have had amputations may still complain of pain in their fingers and toes of the missing limb. This will eventually get better—I hope. The moral to the story, if you have pain get to a dentist.

If you are having pain, get to the dentist. If cold stops the pain, get to the dentist that day or the next day the office is open. If you start swelling, you need to be seen right now. If you cannot get to a dentist, get to a hospital and get on antibiotics. If you are swelling but the pain is less you must be seen that day. This is a true dental emergency and people can die from these infections if they are ignored.

16. Oral surgery

A lot of what I know about oral surgery was self taught on a beachhead in Vietnam

Oral Surgery is a specialty of dentistry. The procedures done by surgeons include extraction of teeth, placing implants, doing bone surgery associated with orthodontic treatment and the biopsy and removal of questionable tissues of the mouth. Some surgeons in some states will go as far as major cancer surgery, and plastic surgery of the face and neck. A few will also do breast augmentation

Extraction of teeth

The removal of teeth that have erupted into the mouth is often done by general dentists. If these teeth protrude through the tissue and if the patient has no complicating medical problems it is more convenient and much less costly to have your general practitioner remove the teeth. If there are potential complications, such as very long or curved roots, broken down crowns, or if your general dentist just prefers to not remove teeth you may be referred to a surgeon.

I want to be asleep

Many people will prefer to go to a surgeon because they want to be asleep for the surgery. You should realize that there are risks to general anesthesia or even IV sedation. Most oral surgery is done with you deeply sedated but not completely under general anesthesia. This is somewhat less risky but it still requires all the monitoring and skill of general anesthesia. You should realize that in almost all cases, the surgeon will also be giving you anesthesia. There will not be an anesthesiologist giving you your anesthesia. No MD surgeon would be allowed to give you general anesthesia and remove your appendix.

The surgeon should stay with you.

The surgery assistant

How about he assistant who is left with you? They may have as little training as a weekend course on how to take blood pressures, how to read a pulse oximeter and write anesthesia records. They are not adequately trained nor is it legal for them to give drugs or treat severe medical emergencies. I would insist and get in writing that the surgeon or an anesthesiologist is in the room the whole time I am asleep under general anesthesia or IV sedation. If I am the patient or if one of my family members is the patient, I would insist on this. They only have one death in 700,000 anesthetic patients, their figures – self reports are notoriously conservative. Death is 100% if it is you or one of your family members.

To read more about anesthesia go to chapter on fear – deep IV sedation general anesthesaia chapter 11.

Why are teeth removed?

Orthodontics

It is sometimes necessary to remove bicuspid teeth to allow more room to rearrange the teeth by an orthodontist. This will usually happen around age 12. Primary, baby teeth, are sometimes removed for orthodontic reasons. By removing primary teeth, permanent teeth can erupt into position earlier. This can be important for the orthodontist. Once in a while, I would find an orthodontist who wanted me to not only remove the baby tooth but also go after the partially formed permanent tooth under the primary tooth. I only had one or two orthodontists who requested this. I stopped referring patients to them because this was much more traumatic for the child than to let the permanent teeth erupt into position and remove them later. It certainly was not the standard and I did not wish to put my child patients through this. An argument could be made that since the child needs the tooth out why not put them to sleep and get it all done? This requires general anesthesia and there are some risks to general anesthesia particularly if it is delivered by the same person doing the surgery. I will discuss this later in this chapter.

Periodontal disease and endo problems

There are a variety of other reasons to remove a tooth. Advanced periodontal disease may have caused the loss of bone support to the point where the tooth is loose and cannot be saved. The nerve of a tooth can die and become infected. If this happens there are two choices, remove the tooth or do a root canal. In general it is much better to do the root canal; however, sometimes this is not possible. The most common reason is because a tooth is a wisdom tooth, the 3rd molar.

Wisdom teeth

It is the belief of much of the population, most dentists, and all oral surgeons that all wisdom teeth, third molars, should be removed, and for the most part, the sooner the better after age 12. Third molars are the tonsils of dentistry. This will be discussed in chapter 17.

Badly broken down teeth

Often patients put off care until there is just not enough tooth left to restore. If decay gets into the nerve, pulp, of the tooth the nerve becomes infected. This infection often leads to extreme pain and sometimes to swelling and fever. It can become life threatening if the infection spreads to the other facial tissues. The answer to the problem is prevention. Get decay taken care of before it get to this point. If you put off treatment or if a nerve dies for other reasons, you have two options: either have the nerve removed and have the nerve chamber filled (a root canal), or have the tooth extracted. It is almost always better to save a tooth but, because of cost, it is not always possible for a patient to afford the root canal. A small percentage of root canals fail, about 3%, and have to be removed. Some teeth will break in such a way that they cannot be saved. Some patients are so apprehensive they will let decay go so long that there simply is not enough tooth structure left to save. Many teeth are lost because of periodontal disease and the loss of bone holding the tooth. If it is not surrounded by good bone, the tooth will become loose and painful and may need to be removed.

What other problems can occur?

It has been suggested to get an x-ray every 5 years or so of impacted teeth to be sure they are not developing a cyst. All teeth develop in a tissue sack. It is possible that this sack can expand. This is a cyst (fluid filled sack). It is not cancer but it can enlarge and cause the loss of bone tissue in the jaw. If you check every 5 years you will pick this up in time to get the problem resolved before there is a major problem. The incidence of these cysts is very low.

Crowding

Get wisdom teeth removed because they will cause your teeth to become crowded. There have been several studies that showed the presence or absence of third molars has nothing to do with crowding of teeth. Teeth tend to have very slight movement when you chew or bite. This will cause some wear. If nothing compensates for this you would end up with space between your teeth. Food would get impacted in these spaces and either decay or gum problems would follow. Our bodies have a way to solve this problem. It is called mesial drift. All our teeth tend to migrate toward the front, midline, of your mouths during life. In this way, the potential space is closed. Our anterior teeth, particularly lowers have a tendency to slightly slip past each other, causing crowding. This has nothing to do with the presence or absence of third molars, however.

You are away

You may be off at college and your wisdom teeth will create problems during finals. This is possible. However, if you do a normal job of brushing and flossing, the chance is very remote. Should it happen, warm rinses and a course of antibiotics should solve the problem until you can get to a surgeon. You may slip and break your ankle but you do not go out and have both legs placed in casts when you go off to college.

You are about to ship out on a round the world sailing adventure where you will be away from land for weeks at a time. In this case, you should have a rather complete medical kit to take care of whatever medical problems you may encounter. Again, a few days of warm rinses and a course of antibiotics should hold you. Is this the unneeded use of antibiotics? Not really, because you truly have an infection. But if the teeth had been removed, you would not have faced the infection. This may or may not be true. There a significant chance of infection after an extraction and the need would be for antibiotics. The incidence of infection is probably about equal after an extraction, as you would have if you left them. Remember, most teeth come in with little in the way of complications other than a little pain and some local swelling until they break through the tissue.

You are going to Mars

You are a member of the team chosen to be first to Mars and will not have a dentist on the space ship with you. This may be a legitimate reason to have them extracted.

Complications – a dry socket

What are the complications of having a 3rd molar removed or for that matter any tooth removed? You can end up with a "dry socket." A dry socket is fairly common particularly for lower wisdom teeth. Normally, after an extraction, a blood clot fills the space where the tooth was. This clot is slowly transformed into soft tissue and, later, bone. If the clot is lost, you are left with a hole in the bone. Food and saliva can get into this hole where it sours. This is irritating to the tissues in the socket and causes a dull pain that can be controlled with analgesics. It also leads to a bad taste that just will not go away.

I have found the easiest control of the taste and pain of a dry socket is to get the patient a plastic syringe and have them rise with warm salt water every hour or so during the day. Some patients also found it was necessary to use Ibuprophen. The good news is the condition goes away in about 14 days if you treat it and 2 weeks if you do nothing. By this time the gum tissue manages to seal up the hole where the tooth was. It may take up to a year for the bone to completely fill in the hole. While the dry socket is uncomfortable, it rarely leads to other complications.

Infection

Once in a while, a tooth, wisdom or otherwise, may be infected. This can lead to swelling of the facial tissue, we call this cellulitis. The patient generally does not feel well and often runs a temperature. Should any of this happen, you need to go to a dentist. On a weekend, if you cannot find your dentist, go to a hospital emergency room. On Monday, find a new dentist with an emergency number.

These infections can lead to death. I know of one where the patient was seen on Friday, Saturday, Sunday, Monday was admitted to a hospital and passed away on Thursday. His tooth was infected with a bacteria that was resistant to any single antibiotic. By the time cultures were done and the appropriate combination was known, it was too late. Fortunately this is very rare.

However, if you have pain in your mouth, your face is swelling, and you are running a temperature, you need to see someone and see them now. This is particularly true if your eye starts to swell closed or the swelling starts to go below your jaw down your neck. Get to a hospital or dentist immediately. Tomorrow is not soon enough.

Extractions are classified

The difficulty of the extraction will affect the incidence of complications, the amount of pain you will have, and the cost. These classifications are used by insurance companies to determine the level of reimbursement for extractions. The classifications are simple first tooth, second tooth, surgical extraction, partial tissue impaction, tissue impaction, partial bony impaction, and full bony impaction.

First tooth refers to needing one tooth removed or a series of teeth. The first tooth costs more because of the set up. The second, third, and forth use the same set up so are less costly to be removed.

Surgical extraction refers to the necessity to peel back tissue and remove bone to get a tooth out. It has nothing to do with a surgeon doing the extraction.

Partial tissue impaction means that part of the tooth is covered by tissue. This tissue must be reflected to get to the tooth. Tissue impaction indicates the tooth is covered by tissue.

Partial boney impaction is a tooth that has tissue and bone covering part of the top of the tooth, occlusal surface.

Full bony impaction means the tooth is completely covered by bone.

There is a tendency by some surgeons to upgrade the difficulty of the extraction. I referred the husband of one of my assistants to a surgeon I trusted. The patient had two very difficult full bony impactions. He also had two very easy erupted third molars. I would call them "gimmeys." He charged the fellow for two full bony impactions and two surgical extractions. The assistant came to me with the bill and asked about why I had told her they would be so easy. I called the surgeon and asked if he might have made a billing error. He said, "No, that was correct." I told him they were very simple extractions that would be out in 10 seconds with no flap or bone removal. He said, "I am very upset you are making this call." I told him I was very upset that I had to make the call. I never referred him another patient. It cost him 12 to 16 wisdom teeth a week; that is, $16,000 TO $20,000 a week in today's dollars. Unfortunately it is very common for surgeons to upgrade the difficulty of extractions."

I had another case where a preauthorization was sent to an insurance company. All 4 thirds were billed as full boney impaction. All were in the mouth through the tissue. I called the office, "I think you sent the wrong x-ray." I always give them the benefit of the doubt.
The receptionist, "No, that is the right x-ray."
Me, "These are not full bony impactions. They have erupted through the tissue."

The receptionist, "We code them all that way."
Me, "Ma'am your dentist is committing fraud."
The receptionist, "How could that be? He has never seen this x-ray."
Me, "Who looked at the x-ray and decided these were full bony impactions?"
The receptionist, "I did."
Me, "Ma'am, are you a dentist?
The receptionist, "Do you think I would be answering the phone if I were the dentist?"
Me, "Ma'am, you are practicing dentistry, if you are reading x-rays. Your dentist could lose his license for letting you do that."
The receptionist, "How could that be? This patient has never been in the office."
Me, "I'll tell you what, I will send back these x-rays. Have the dentist read the x-rays and resubmit the claim."
The moral to the story, be careful if you are getting surgery done in Anchorage Alaska or anywhere else.

What is orthognathic surgery?

Sometimes, if the upper or low jaw does not develop adequately or develops too much it may be impossible to get front teeth together to chew. It also may mean that it is impossible to get good results with orthodontic treatment. To resolve this problem, the lower jaw may be sectioned and moved forward or back. Sometimes, it is necessary to do the same to the upper jaw. This is major surgery and can have serious complications.

I found some orthodontic / oral surgery teams almost always found it necessary to do this. It was like the old west where gun slingers notched their six shooters after every encounter. I think the orthodontists were notching their mirrors with each case.

When I started practice, no one needed this because the surgery technique was not commonly taught. Within a few years, it seemed everyone needed it. I did notice that some orthodontists rarely suggest this procedure, so I referred my patients to them. If a patient found an orthodontist who was suggesting this, I would council them about the potential complication and refer them for a second opinion.

Some cases can not be done without it. But these are extremes, Jay Leno, Andy Gump type profiles.

Oral cancer surgery

Some surgeons do cancer surgery. Fortunately, oral cancer is rather rare. Unfortunately, it often is not discovered until it is advanced and it is difficult to treat. It is a minor part of the whole picture of oral surgery. Oral cancer in the past was a disease of old, undernourished patients who smoked heavily, several packs a day, and drank large amounts of alcohol each day.

In the last 10 years, oral cancer is being seen in the under 40 crowd who neither drinks or smokes. They are well nourished. Human papilloma virus (HPV-16 and 18) is the cause of genital wards that can lead to cervical cancers. We are now seeing these lesions in the oral cavity and they are leading to oral cancer in this younger group.

The bad news is the 5 year survival rate of oral cancer is about 50% and it has not changed much in the last 40 years, while most other cancers have improved survival rates due to early detection and better treatments. Oral cancers, in their early stages, are very difficult to detect and, consequently, they tend to be found in their more advanced stages. There are new devices now being marketed that may help with early detection of oral cancers.

Other cosmetic surgery

Some surgery training programs go beyond what was traditionally considered the perview of oral surgeons, treating the hard and soft tissues of the oral cavity. There are surgeons doing nose jobs, eyelid lifts, facial skin treatments, and breast reductions and augmentation. It depends on the State regulations where they practice.

My suggestion, if you need plastic surgery, go to a plastic surgeon. If you have nose jobs go to an ENT doctor or plastic surgeon. This is a turf war. I watched as an anesthesia resident took out third molars calling them Odontomas, a tooth tumor. I watched Plastic Surgery residents set broken jaws. The teeth usually did not mesh very well when they were done. I also saw oral surgeon residents try to do plastic and ENT procedures. It is better if you go to the specialist who spends all their time working in their own area.

Osteonecrosis of the jaw (ONJ)

There is a group of drugs being used that is causing concern for dentists. This problem first came to my attention early in 2006. We heard many opinions over the year and it appears it may not be as big a problem as we once thought; at least the risk of problems is quite low. It is an issue you should be aware of, however, particularly if you are on one of the drugs.

The bisphosphonates

The bisphosphonates are used to stop the progression of osteoporosis. The drugs now used are Fosamax, Didronel, Boniva, Aredia, Actonel, Skelid or Zometa It is becoming very common for women approaching and in menopause to be on one of these drugs. The drugs are also used as IV treatment for some forms of cancer. They stop the process of bone remodeling that is believed to contribute to bone loss. This, however, also makes it harder for bone to heal after dental surgery.

We added the following question to our medical history:

> *Do you have osteoporosis or have you taken the following: Fosamax, Didronel, Boniva, Aredia,*

Actonel, Skelid or Zometa? (These are drugs used to treat osteoporosis. They can cause major problems for extractions)   YES / NO.

Why is this important?

If you have dental surgery that involves your bone, such as tooth extractions or periodontal surgery, your bone may not heal. This leaves an open sore in your mouth that will not heal and may never heal.

Fortunately, it is very rare if you are taking the oral drugs. It is much more common for those with cancer who must have the IV drugs.

Can you just stop the drugs?

Can you just stop the drugs if you need dental surgery? The half-life of these drugs is about 7 years. If you stopped the drug, in 7 years half the drug effect is gone. In 14 years 3/4 of the effect is gone. One study showed that if the drugs were stopped the defect would heal in 9 to 12 months.

The drugs are important because by slowing or stopping bone loss there is less chance of breaking a hip or having spine problems. A high number of elderly die after breaking a hip. So if you need the drugs, keep taking them.

Risk of complications with oral drugs is very low

The risk of problems for those on the oral

medication is very low. The risk of complications from a broken hip is very high. If you are taking the IV form for cancer, you cannot stop. **If the drugs are needed we simply must live with the possible complications.**

17. Third molars—wisdom teeth

Prophylactic extractions of 3rd molars is assigning disease state to a non-diseased condition.

If you ask people on the street about wisdom teeth, everyone has heard of them, but no one knows where they got their name. Actually, this seems to be the only tooth people call by a name. But why the name? Whoever called it that anyway? No one seems to know, but it probably has to do with them coming into the mouth in our late teens early 20s when we are at our smartest. Wisdom teeth, the farthest back teeth #1, #16, #17 and #32 are also known as 3rd molars.

They have not affected our evolution

Mankind evolved for the first half million years without having wisdom teeth removed. It was only after the development of local anesthesia and, later, the use of general anesthesia that it became necessary, in vogue, to remove these. Some of our ancestors suffered because of these teeth and some probably died of untreated infections due to these teeth. However, the numbers were too small to alter the evolution of man. While it is true that some people never develop these teeth they are in the minority. Had third molars been a species-threatening problem we would expect that the incidence of missing wisdom teeth would be greater, or there would be fewer people who had problems. The worst-case scenario would have been the extinction of our species. Obviously none of this happened.

Surgeons will tell you wisdom teeth should all be removed because they may cause problems when they erupt into the mouth. If we did that to every tooth that causes some pain and inflammation when erupting, we would remove all the teeth.

About 10% will have a problem

Most people have third molars erupt through the gum tissue into their mouths between 16 and 25 years of age. Only about ten percent of the population will have problems with wisdom teeth other then the expected discomfort of these breaking through the gum tissue, to take their proper position in the mouth. This may be a more recognized problem because this process of teething happens to adults. We pay little attention to kids who are teething as it is expected and happens when they are much younger. If we removed all teeth that caused some pain or swelling as they came through the tissue, none of us would have any teeth.

About 10% of third molars cause problems, which is about the same percentage for gallbladders and appendix surgery, but we do not prophylactically remove gall bladders or appendixes. No other major medical or dental specialty except perhaps plastic surgery makes so much money from so little pathology.

The problems of wisdom teeth

The problems of wisdom teeth come in several flavors. The may be uncomfortable when they erupt and then settle down. They may never come in. They may be sideways; they can then destroy the bone of the next tooth forward in the mouth, the second molar. The tissue around the wisdom tooth may become infected if the tooth only comes part way in.

Some surgeons and orthodontists will tell you they will cause crowding of your other teeth. There have been several studies that show this is not true. They will tell you is it less painful to do early. This is not true. It is safer to remove early. This is not true.

Problems in old age

Several reasons have been suggested for the prophylactic removal of these teeth including removing them at a convenient time to prevent future problems. It has included getting them out while you are young and healthy so they do not cause problems when you are old and have other medical problems that might be exacerbated because of the trauma of the extraction—you are 80 years old, have a bad heart, and it is now a life threatening procedure.

The studies say leave them

There was a study of 54 other studies that looked at the chance of problems later versus the problems of having the teeth removed prophylactically. They did not show a greater number of problems by waiting nor did they show more problems for the few elderly who needed to have them removed at a later date. The conclusion was that, if you are over 35, there are fewer problems by leaving them alone than by having them removed. In fact, there was no evidence that the older patient who had third molars removed, if they caused problems at a later date, had any more complications or suffered more from the extractions than younger patients.

Should all wisdom teeth be removed

Should all wisdom teeth be removed? In America it is almost a right of passage of growing up. You have your wisdom teeth removed about the same time you get your driver's license. This costs about 2.5 billion dollars every year and keeps some 8,000 oral surgeons busy. Is it wise to do this? Or even necessary?

In a word, no

Generally, the answer is no. If you were going to spend a year in a third world country where there were no dentists and it looked like your teeth might erupt during that time, I might recommend that you have them out. If you were selected for a 5 years mission to Mars, I would recommend you have them out. There are no dentists between here and there. If your child was going to be in an area where there were dentists when they go to college or start working, I would not recommend it. You can always have them out if and when they become a problem.

If only pathologic third molars were removed, we would save close to 80% in cost and unnecessary pain. It causes each patient an average of about 3 days of pain, close to 3,000,000 cumulative lost days of school or work for our population. About one in one hundred are left partially or permanently numb from the surgery. A few unlucky ones will have permanent numbness to the whole lower arch (lower half of their face) for life.

Incidence of problems used to frighten people:

Carcinoma, cancer of 3rd molar is so rare that there are no statistics.

Cysts, sacks, around teeth; less than 1% of 3rd molars have cysts. This is based on x-rays that show cysts that are greater than 2 mm.
Damage to adjacent teeth; Root resorption 5%

Crowding of anterior teeth—no evidence in two JADA papers. Crowding of incisors occur as a consequence of anterior component of occlusal force if the arch of anterior jaw is too small for alignment of all the teeth.

What is the risk

If you are a male and live to be 80 years old, you will have a good chance of getting prostate cancer. If you are a female, you have a 1 in 7 chance of having breast cancer. However, no one in their right mind has the prostate or breast removed from our 16 year olds just in case a cancer of that organ happens. Does it make sense to remove all the third molars when only about 10% are ever a problem? If they do become a problem they can be removed at that time. I do not think this makes any sense at all. In fact, in most countries, our custom of removing wisdom teeth is considered just as shocking and barbaric as removing a healthy prostate to prevent cancer in the future.

So how do you tell the legitimate cases of wisdom teeth problems from the automatic wholesale recommendation of wisdom teeth removal? Let's look at some examples.

Leave healthy teeth alone

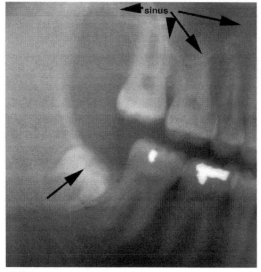

Figure 17.1

This x-ray shows a large sinus dropping below the level of root tip of the upper 1st molar, the second tooth from the back; the back molar is a second molar, and if there was a wisdom tooth above, it would be a 3rd molar. If you are confused go on to the next section. Go on to the next section even if you do understand this.

The lower wisdom tooth had not yet developed a root but is facing the right direction to erupt into place (see arrow). It may erupt into place given time. There is no need to do anything to this tooth

These teeth will probably erupt

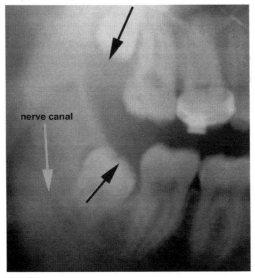

Figure 17.2

In this x-ray, both upper and lower third molars have the potential to erupt into a useful position. The nerve channel is at the base of the lower third molar. There is a risk of removing such a tooth. The nerve can be injured during the extraction. Should this happen this child could permanently be numb on this side of his low jaw including half the lower lip. This makes drinking liquids difficult and kissing only half as much fun. Besides, since both teeth are positioned properly, there is no need for an extraction.

These teeth need to be removed

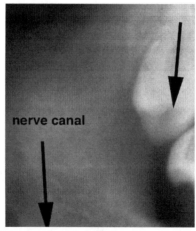

Figure 17.3 These teeth need to be removed.

This x-ray shows the upper and lower third molars angled in such a direction that they will never erupt into a functional position and have a significant risk of doing damage to the tooth they have come up against. The root of the lower molar is in close proximity to the nerve canal. There is a high risk of damaging the nerve when this tooth is removed. Both of these teeth should be removed. If the lower is not removed, no bone will form to support that back root of the tooth in front of it. If the tooth is taken out early there is a chance you will get a bone fill. If you wait until the patient is an adult and then remove the tooth there is little chance of getting bone to fill the defect. There is a risk of getting a permanent numbness, but you need to take this risk because the risk of leaving this tooth is greater, and eventually it will need to be removed with even a greater chance of problems.

Here is the patient several years later

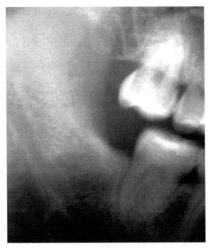

Figure 17.4 Here is the patient several years later.

This is that same patient several years after the upper and lower wisdom teeth were removed. The extraction has been done properly. Bone has filled in the holes where the teeth were, No damage was done to the nerve or the teeth they were up against.

Four on the floor or just the offending teeth

If there is a need to remove the wisdom teeth, should all 4 be removed at one time? This really depends on the problem and what the other thirds look like. It probably does not make much sense to remove them all if only one is a problem, unless it is very clear the others will also be problems in the future. If the tissue over a third molar becomes swollen or infected, get rid of the molar. If it is causing the tooth in front of it to be damaged, get rid of the molar. If it is just there, I would wait and see if it ever becomes a problem. Chances are very good it never will.

3rd molar removal is SURGERY

Remember, removing wisdom teeth is surgery. It can cause some problems, including permanent numbness, infection, pain and, every now and then, someone will die of these complications or the complications of general anesthesia. There was a child in Texas who had third molars removed with sedation and died as a complication of the sedation, obesity, and an undiagnosed heart problem. It has been estimated that one in every 700,000 people put to sleep in oral surgery offices die. This is a small risk unless you happen to be the one.

Orthodontist will suggest removal

Orthodontists will often suggest a child's 3rd molars be removed. Some believe they can push on the teeth in front of them and those teeth push on the next teeth until the front teeth become crowded. There has been good research to show this does not happen. It was used by orthodontists for years to explain why an orthodontic case became crowded after the treatment was completed. The research looked at two groups of orthodontic patients: those who had their 3rd molars removed and those who still had there 3rd molars. Neither group had a greater percentage of relapse, failure of the orthodontic treatment.

Finally, if the bone is lost around the tooth due to periodontal disease or infection from a dead nerve or infection from the gingival tissue, the tooth may need to be removed. Even decay is a reasonable reason to remove a 3rd molar. Just having third molars is not a reason to have them removed.

> I got a call from an orthodontist. She said, "Who do you use for 3rd molar extractions? I think Joe should have his out." I responded, "They look to me like they may come in OK. Why take them out?" She said, "Well, I think they should come out. They may cause crowding." To which I said, "you know there was research that showed that is not caused by having 3rd." "Well, I think they

should come out. I will tell his parents they should come out." "That is OK. I too will talk to them. They can decide what they want done."

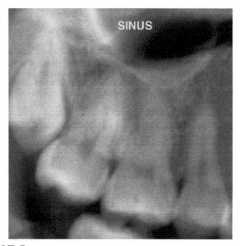

Figure 17.5

Your jaws

You upper jaw, or maxilla, holds the upper teeth. The bone above the roots of the posterior teeth also houses the maxillary sinuses. Some sinuses are even larger than this patient. These are air-filled holes in the bone that communicate with our nasal passages. They make our heads lighter than it would be if it were solid bone. They also tend to warm and humidify the air we inhale. The sinuses also make our voices sound different. They make our voices resonate.

The first notice most of us pay to our sinuses is when they become infected. These sinus infections can be very frustrating to cure. This condition is a problem for medical doctors rather than dentists.

> *Now and again a sinus infection will feel like a toothache. I was called to the office one morning at 3AM. I took x-rays, did all the tests I could think of, and I could not figure out which tooth was causing the pain. I am not the most cognitive creature when I am awakened in the middle of the night. I finally told the patient I would numb her up with a long-acting local anesthesia. She should go home and get a good night's sleep. I would do the same and I would see her at 10AM when we both would be thinking more effectively. She did not show up at 10Am or 11AM. If you get me up in the middle of the night, you really should come in for your appointment. At about this time, my receptionist came to me and told me the patient had just called. She was at her physician's and had been diagnosed with a sinus infection. She was not suffering from a tooth problem after all.*

Sinuses may be an issue

Sinuses can cause dental problems as well, because the roots of molars and bicuspids often are covered by only a very thin layer of bone and, sometimes, even no bone, just the membrane lining the sinus. If these teeth need to be extracted, it is possible to get a hole into the sinus that can be difficult to close.

> *One such case was reported where every time the patient drank coffee it came out his nose. A dentist had extracted a tooth and got a sinus perforation that he either did not realize was there or simply hoped would close on its own.*

Unfortunately, for the dentist and the patient it did not close. No this was not me.

I always warn my surgery patients that this can happen. When extracting teeth, it is possible to lose a root or tooth into the sinus area. This happened to me once in 40 years. I lost a piece of root about 3 mm long 1/32 of an inch. I sent the patient to an Otolaryngologist (Ear, Nose, and Throat - ENT Dr.). He said it would never be a problem and suggested it be left alone.

Orthoganathic surgery

Fortunately, these discrepancies can be corrected with orthoganathic surgery, where the lower jaw is sectioned and either moved back or forward. In the most severe cases the upper jaw may also be advanced or retracted.

Problems with orthoganathic surgery

The bad news is this is major surgery with all the risks of general anesthesia. In rare cases when the upper jaw has been sectioned, the section that has been moved can lose blood supply. This causes the bone to die, and a large section of bone and the front teeth can be lost. Needless to say, this is a very major problem that is impossible to reverse and very difficult to repair with a prosthetic device.

It is also possible for such facial surgery to cause numbness in one or both sides of the lower jaw, including the lips. This can be permanent and it feels much like the sensation of being numbed to have dentistry done on the lower teeth, only the numbness never goes away. It is hard to drink liquids because you cannot feel your lower lip. Nor is there as much pleasure from kissing, as I have indicated before.

The discrepancy in size of the upper and lower jaws can lead to teeth crowding, which in turn necessitates orthodontic treatment, or braces. In America, it simply is not acceptable to have crooked teeth. However, there are some exceptions. Jay Leno, David Letterman, Condoleezza Rice, Terry Thomas, and Tom Cruise have all done well despite not having perfect teeth. For the rest of us mere mortals, it has become the norm to have braces when in middle school or high school in the US. This is not so true in the rest of the world.

Health Advantage Summary

1. If you have teeth, do everything you can to keep them. Nothing we do is half as good as what you started with.
2. Clean and floss your teeth regularly. Ideally you would brush and floss after every meal, but at least brush twice a day and floss every evening. If you will not floss, brush even more. If you will not brush more or floss, use a fluoride gel— even on adult teeth.
3. If you have a dental problem, always ask what will happen if you do not seek treatment.

4. It is your option to have a perfect smile, with white straight teeth. It is also your option to not go through extensive, expensive makeovers. Not everyone has to have the same smile. Really.

5. Consider your medical status as a factor in your treatment.

18. The culture of orthodontics

In America, if you do not have straight white teeth, you are sub-human

The explosion of aesthetics – braces – orthodontics

The American model is that we all have perfectly aligned teeth that are the color of chicklets. Nowhere in the world is this true to the extent it is here. The theory is you will be more successful, more self-confident, more loved if you have a perfect smile. To a certain extent this is true. There have been studies that show tall, slim, good looking people with straight teeth make more money.

Many examples of success with less than perfect teeth

However, there a plenty of examples of people with less prefect smiles are successful. The former CEO of Boeing had two front teeth that a 747 could fly between. Jay Leno has a chin that sticks out well beyond the ideal. David Letterman also has a large gap between his front teeth. The Late Terry Thomas, and English actor, could almost store his tongue between his front teeth. June Carter-Cash had front teeth that were so far forward only Mister Ed's front teeth were more prominent, but June could really sing. Reese Witherspoon who played June in the movie, "Walk the line," is just the reverse: her lower jaw is much larger then her upper jaw but she is none the less a very beautiful woman and has a wonderful voice. Even Tom Cruse has a defect. His midline is off almost a whole tooth. You never see a straight on photo of him for this reason. All of these folks are quite successful even with their defect. What do all these people have in common? They were very successful and needed orthodontic intervention. Who knows just how much more successful they might have been if they had a perfect smile.

Figure 18.1 You will notice that the middle of Tom's face, the left line. Is much different than the middle of his smile, right line.

Orthognathic surgery

About 30 years ago, oral surgeons started doing orthognathinc surgery to correct mismatched jaw sizes. Where the lower jaw or upper jaw is much larger or smaller than ideal, it may not be possible to move teeth with braces and achieve ideal or even good results. Surgeons can section the upper or lower or both jaws and reposition the segments to come up with a more ideal result. In some cases, this is the only way to get an ideal result. It may be necessary in some severe cases to even be able to bring the teeth together to adequately chew. This is major surgery but it may be necessary.

Orthognathic surgery became so common it was almost as if it was being done to establish bragging rights as to how many cases you were involved with if you were an orthodontist or oral surgeon. Yes, the orthodontics was faster if the patient had orthognathic surgery. Yes, sometimes you could get better results. Yes, the cases may have had better long-term results. In many cases this could have been done with braces with no surgery. However, it was expeditious to do it with surgery. The orthodontist still did the orthodontics but a surgeon was not on the team to do the surgery. The cost more than doubled. Orthognathic surgery is very major surgery with difficult challenges for the anesthesiologist. We are now seeing some surgeons doing this surgery in their offices, some are even giving their own anesthesia for these cases. This is major surgery and to do both is really pushing the envelope. A medical surgeon cannot take out your appendix and do the anesthesia. Appendectomies are far less complex than most jaw resections.

A new orthodontist was out introducing himself to local dentists. One invited him back to the treatment area. There was a 40 year old with crowded front teeth.

The "fine aesthetic dentist" explained how with oral sedation he was going to crown 14 upper and 14 lower teeth that day. The patient would go home with a beautiful smile in temporaries and would get the final crowns in two weeks getting an even more beautiful smile.

The dentist asked, "Can you do that as an orthodontist?" The orthodontist left the office shaking his head.

Why was the orthodontist concerned? The cost of 28 crowns would be 8 to 9 times more costly than orthodontics, or braces. ($28,000 to $33,000 for the crowns vs.$3-$4,000 for braces).

After orthodontics, the patient would need to sleep with a retainer to prevent relapse but would have "virgin" teeth, that is, teeth that are structurally in exactly the same state as Mother Nature gave the patient.

Of the 28 crowned teeth, we can conservatively estimate that at a minimum 2 or 3 would need a root canal in the next 10 years. If the crowns were done in the new all porcelain materials that number could double because more tooth structure would need to be removed to do the all porcelain crowns.

In addition, even if the dentist was very good (which is doubtful if the dentist suggested this treatment), the whole case would need to be redone at some point, perhaps in 12 to 17 years. Even more teeth would die at that time.

If the dentist's surgical skills were reflected in the decision to crown all these teeth, the redo might be needed in as little as 5 to 10 years.

So spend $50,000 to $60,000 for crowns or $3,000 for orthodontics. This is not an extreme example. It is being done all the time. Patients of some less *scrupulous dentists choose the crowns because they don't want to sport the unsightly braces and they want an "instant smile." The really sad part is orthodontics like this case can be done with the invisible techniques; it just takes a little longer.*

What happens if I say no

One should always ask what happens if I do not do this surgery. What are the risks of the surgery? What is the chance of life threatening complications or death? Remember the chance of death is low, but it is 100% if it is you. In my mouth, which needed orthodontics, I would not submit myself to this risk, particularly if the job could be done with conventional braces.

Some orthodontists almost always recommend this surgery. Others almost never recommend it. I stopped referring my patients to those who seemed to use it an unreasonable amount.

Invisiline

Recently, a new technique has been developed to do orthodontics. Models are made of the patient's mouth and sent to a company that scans them into a computer and generates what looks like a series of bite guards each being slightly different from the preceding one. By placing pressure on teeth you can tip them into position. By changing each appliance just a little you can move the teeth a bit and then go to the next appliance that moves the tooth a little further. By going through a series of appliances, you can align teeth in mouths that are not that complex. No wires, brackets, or bands are necessary. However, this technique is limited to only simple cases.

Is orthodontics necessary

Is it necessary to have straight teeth? Many will say yes, particularly if you ask an orthodontist. As a teenager, I would have given anything to have straight teeth. We just could not do it. I have done OK. Would I have done better? Maybe. Would I have been a better person? I doubt it. It certainly would have made you even more of a stud.

VI. The nonspecialties

HERMAN®

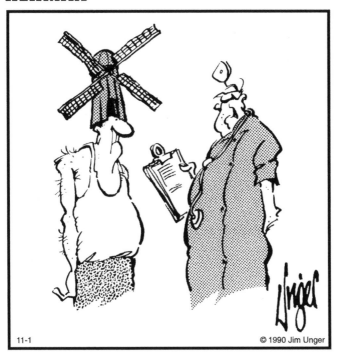

11-1 © 1990 Jim Unger

**"I think I've discovered why you
keep grinding your teeth."**

19. The Temporomandibular Joint – TMJ or why I grind my teeth

Most of us will have sore chewing muscles at some time in our life

Neural muscular dentistry

Your lower jaw or mandible is U-shaped, and your tongue fits in the middle of the U. The lower jawbone is denser than the upper arch because there is much less bone and the bone must be stronger to make up for the lack of bulk.

The lower jaw is attached to the upper jaw by the temporomandibular joint, TMJ. There are a number of muscles attached to the mandible that allow us to chew, talk, move our jaw, make faces, etc. When under stress, many of us will clench our teeth by tightening these muscles. This can cause wear on our teeth. It is even possible to break teeth in this way, although fortunately that's rare.

We all have a unique joint, the temporomandibular joint, TMJ. As you open your mouth, the TMJ first acts like a hinge. As you open further, it slides forward. There is a cushioning disk that normally slides with the lower half of the joint. If this disk pops out of position you can hear the pop. Roughly 1/3 of the population pops when they open their mouths. This is nothing to be concerned about unless it causes pain. Of course we would like you to be able to open your mouth pain free. The good news for sufferers is this tends to be a problem of young adults under 35 years of age. It also seems to go away as we get older. Unfortunately, it is about 7 times more common in women than in men.

TMJ

Many, if not most, people have facial pain, headaches, muscle pain, and joint pain at some point in their lives. These very real and very unpleasant symptoms are sometimes lumped into TMJ. This is a misnomer as we all have TMJ. TMJ is temporomandibular joint, or the jaw joint found just forward of your ear. Put your fingers about half an inch in front of your ear and open your mouth. The bump you feel moving is the mandibular portion of your TMJ.

In fact we all have TMJ, temporomandibular joints. The painful muscle is more properly called MPD, for myofacial pain dysfunction. You never find people in nursing homes holding their jaws. They might hold knees, ankles, elbows, shoulders, yes, but not their jaws. Unfortunately, for women, they suffer 7 times more problems than men. This is because men drive women crazy.

Problems can happen when there is a disharmony in the size of the upper and lower jaws. Some examples of this are Jaws in James Bond movies and Jay Leno . You can clearly see that the lower jaw is larger than the upper jaw. The opposite problem can be the other way, commonly known as Andy Gump or weak chin retrognathia.

The experts cannot agree

Various methods of treatment have been suggested. There must, at any one time, be a dozen experts lecturing on how to solve this problem. I once took a 10 day course on the problem one afternoon a week for 10 weeks. A variety of experts from a dental school presented a very complete discussion of all aspects of this joint. The conclusion was the less you do the better. The patient will get better if left alone. There are some things that can help. Using anti-inflammatory drugs helps. There are some simple physical therapy exercises that can help and bite guards will often help.

Do not let anyone put anything in your jaw joint, TMJ

Do not under any circumstances let someone inject anything into the joint. It is common for some to inject steroids into this joint. The joint is very small, and entering it with a needle will cause some damage. The steroids are potent painkillers and the joint will feel better for a while but it tends to get worse after this. Never, under any circumstances, let someone put an arthroscope into the joint. This will tend to leave you in pain the rest of your life. The joint will feel better for a while because of the nerves that are cut getting the scope in place and the fact that steroids are usually placed at the same time.

Open or close your bite

Others suggest you get all your teeth crowned to open your bite. Still others suggest doing it to close the bite. Both work and both fail and both are very costly. I learned to school patients to adjust the shape of their teeth so they closed with their lower jaw as far back as possible. I am not at all comfortable with my jaw in this position. They chose this position as we could reproduce it as it is the only place where the jaw is stable and we can get back to by manipulating the jaw. Very few people actually chew here, however.

The neural muscular approach

Another group hooks you up to an electronic stimulator to determine just what the correct position is. They also use sensors to see just how your jaw moves when you chew and make recommendations from these records. This is a real process. They place electrodes on the back of your neck and over your jaw joint. Minor electrical current twitches the muscles in this area. This supposedly places your jaw in exactly the best place for it. However, I am a little skeptical that this is exactly the right place to apply the current.

Another plan uses a set of glasses with a grid of wire attached with magnetic sensors. A magnet is glued to your lower front teeth, and then you chew. The sensors show on an oscilloscope just how your jaw moves. If there is an abnormal tracing then they grind your teeth or place crowns to get rid of the abnormality. Is this the correct approach? Who knows, but the technology is impressive. Some experts will tell you it is bogus.

Should you use a bite guard while doing sports and sleeping

No one really knows the correct answer. For some people, anything works; for others, nothing works. The one universal is the recommendation of some sort of bite guard to be worn when sleeping. Most of us clench and/or grind our teeth some when we sleep. The question is, what is the proper bite guard? Many are similar to athletic mouth guards. All athletes of any sport with a potential for contact should wear one of these protective devices. Many of my patients have great results from simply using one of these to sleep in.

Bite guards galore

There are at least 10 different forms of bite guards recommended by the experts— hard ones, soft ones, combinations of hard and soft ones, posterior guards, anterior guards, snore guards (at least 5 varieties), full contact guards, NTI guards, guards developed with electronic stimulation. You make them or we make them. In fact, if you sleep with a pencil between your teeth, it would probably work; however, it would probably fall out and poke your eye out. A good place to start is to make an athletic guard yourself. If this works, go with it. If not, you should talk to your dentist.

DO NOT HAVE TMJ SURGERY (YES I AM SHOUTING)

Many of these patients with joint pain are chronic pain patients. They go from dentist to dentist with little in the way of results. The unlucky ones have someone do surgery. I have reviewed cases where these patients had 10 and 12 surgeries on their TMJs; getting worse after each surgery. They come with a bag full of various bite guards. They need to be seen by an oral medicine specialist. There are oral medicine specialists in most large cities and at all dental schools. These are specialists who have had several years of advanced training in a full time residency in a dental school. Do not be fooled by self-proclaimed TMJ experts, oral pain specialists, or TMJ surgery specialists. Find a specialist in Oral Medicine.

When the experts cannot agree, look out

Almost all adults will at one time or another experience facial pain. We occasionally sleep wrong, suffer stress, clench our teeth, or bite too hard; all these can cause facial pain. I have heard at least 10 different experts describe techniques to deal with this problem. Each one had a different method of treating this. Some pushed using very expensive imaging equipment to see how your jaws moved. Needless to say, they sold the equipment. Once they saw how your jaw moved, they would crown all your teeth to make your jaw move more smoothly. Others suggest you should have all your teeth adjusted until they mesh like the gears of a new Italian sports car. Others felt this was wrong. You should have all your teeth capped so they could make them mesh like a new German touring car. Still others have suggested they would make you bite guards that only touched the back teeth, or only the front teeth. Some wanted bite guards for both the upper and lower arches. Some felt the guards had to be hard plastic, others favored soft cushioning plastic, or some combination of both. There has been at least one study that showed all these approaches worked, but no better than a placebo device that did not change how your teeth come together.

The NTI is here

In the late 1990s, a new device hit the market. It is a simple plastic device that fits over the front upper 4 teeth. This is known as an NTI device. It is reported to cure migraine headaches and all matter of facial pain. It even has FDA approval. This approval, however, is no guarantee it works. It merely indicates the device is safe to use. I looked at the original research that was presented to the FDA. They looked at all forms of oral facial pain and how it was affected by wearing the device. One week one form of pain would respond better, the next week it would be worse but a different form of pain might be better. Try as I might, I simply could not find a trend. The graphs simply were all over the paper. Not quite as chaotic as a seismograph of an earthquake, but not a clear trend either.

Some dentists and patients find it works

Still, some dentists have been using this device to cure all forms of pain. If rubbing bat guano on your earlobes works, go for it. If the NTI works, all the better for you. Pain is bad. But I would be careful about taking your headache to a dentist first. Some forms of brain cancer, brain tumors, strokes, subdural hematomas or blood leaking into the cranial cavity, blood clots in the brain, and various other brain injuries can cause a headache. Have a diagnosis first to be sure your pain is not a sign of a potential life threatening problem. If all is well except for your pain, any of the aforementioned devices may help. There simply is not enough research to say which is best. I tried 10 of these devices on patients and staff who had diagnosed migraines. It did not help a single person. Of course I am such a skeptic I did not describe these devices as an absolute cure so they saw no placebo response.

20. What are implants?

"I am having so much fun chewing with these implants, I may have to sue you, because I am going to get fat."

The problem of a lost tooth

When a tooth is lost, you are left with a space. In most cases that tooth should be replaced. If it is not replaced the adjacent teeth will tend to tip into the space. The tooth in the arch opposing space will tend to over erupt into the space. If the space is up front it will be noticeable and there are more jokes about the IQ of people with missing teeth than we have time for here.

> *Question: What do you have if you have 32 people from Appalachia, Oklahoma, Arkansas, Detroit, etc (insert the group you wish to insult)? Answer: A complete set of teeth. (Is there anyone I did not insult?)*

Will you die if you do not get a tooth replaced?

No, but we were taught in dental school that most if not all missing teeth should be replaced.

> *I had a patient who was missing a back tooth. I explained how it was important to replace it. I explained how teeth would tip and shift. I explained how the adjacent teeth would be stronger splinted together with a bridge.*

She asked me how long all this would take. I explained what I had been taught; that within 5 years there would be major changes in her bite and the alignment of teeth.

She asked how bad it was now. I told her that everything looked good now; but that would change, as she got older. She said it was strange, because she had lost that tooth twenty-six years before. Clearly she was not having any of the changes I had been taught to expect. Maybe in the next 26 years they would start to shift.

In general missing teeth should be replaced

How can a missing tooth be replaced? The classic option is a bridge. To do a bridge the teeth on either side of the space are crowned and a fake tooth is suspended between the two crowns. This requires trimming down the two adjacent teeth. We really do not like to do this if the two teeth are virgin, have never had a crown or a filling. In the past we did not have a choice as a bridge or removable partial denture were the only options

The partial denture is removable. The partial uses metal clasps around the adjacent teeth to hold it in place. It has to be removed and cleaned every time you eat because it tends to collect food. The food, if not removed, will cause the clasped teeth to decay. It also has to have a metal framework that clasps teeth on both sides of the arch. In short it is a lot of appliance to get use to.

I have always told patients who were getting a partial that the day I insert it, they will hate it. It will feel a lot like I slipped a horseshoe into their mouths. You must keep it in your mouth for three weeks removing it only to clean it. After three weeks it will start to feel strange when it is not in your mouth. If you start wearing it in your pocket or the dresser drawer at home you will never get used to it. It does you no good if you do not learn to wear it.

If the missing tooth is the last tooth or, heaven forbid, the last two teeth in an arch you have no choice to do to a partial or to hand one fake tooth off two crowns that were soldered together on the teeth forward of the space. These are known as cantilever bridges and do not work well.

Enter the Implant

In the 1950s and 1960s subperiosteal implants were done to help people with dentures that simply did not work. The patient would be numbed. An incision would be made along the crest of the ridge the denture sat on from the back right to the back left. The tissues would be peeled away much like you peel an orange. This exposed the underlying bond. An impression, mold, of the bone would be taken and the tissues would be sutured back together.

A plaster model would be poured in the mold and a framework would be made that covered the bone with a few holes for screws. Once this was done, the tissue was again peeled back.

The framework would be screwed in place and the tissue would be sutured back. There would be 4 posts that extended from the framework through the tissue. The denture would be attached to these posts.

The patients love these once they have recovered from the surgery. Their dentures were tight for the first time in years. The problem was that with time the gum tissue can grow down around the posts and surround the whole framework and it will become loose. Hopefully, the patient was old enough when the implant was placed that this never happens before the patient is ready to quit chewing.

Blade vent implants

In the late 1970s, we saw the introduction of the blade vent implant. The problem was we knew these would last 5 years but most were lost by ten years. I did have one that lasted 17 years but that was unusual.

Branemark implants

Next we saw a system that came from Sweden. It looks like a bolt with no head. An incision was made to expose a small area of bone. A round hole was drilled into the bone of the upper or lower jaw. The implant was screwed down even with the top of the bone and the gum tissue was sutured over the implant. Six to nine months later the implant was uncovered and a post was screwed into the implant that came through the tissue. A crown was placed on this post. The failure rate of this is probably not greater than 5% over twenty years. They work. They probably are more long lasting than bridges. Some smart people these Swedes.

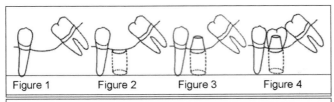

| Figure 1 | Figure 2 | Figure 3 | Figure 4 |

Figure 1 A tooth was lost and the molar is tipping.
Figure 2. A hole is drilled in the bone.
Figure 3. An implant has been placed and the post is in place coming through the gum tissue.
Figure 4. A crown has been place replacing the missing tooth.

Figure 20.1

The biggest problem is the 6 to 9 month wait for the bone to integrate the implant into the bone. The other is the cost. The average implant costs about the same as 3 crowns. In addition, you need to place a crown so from space to crown costs about what 4 crowns would cost. If you need three or four or, heaven forbid, 5 implants, you are talking about really big money. People have given up dentures by having many implants placed and then crowns on these implants. The cost of such cases can top $50,000. Many people will pay this for a car that they only keep for 4 or 5 years but may be reluctant to put that same money in their mouths.

Mini-implants

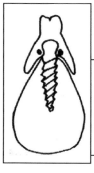

A denture sits on a ridge of the lower arch. The denture is secured in position by a mini implant attached by an O-ring

Figure 20.2   A mini implant

It can be a challenge to keep a denture in while implants are healing. Someone decided to place small implants as a temporary device to hold the denture in place. These are about the size and shape of a small wood screw but made of titanium. They are about 12 to 15 mm long and 2 mm in diameter. A small hole is drilled into the bone and the implant is screwed into the hole. This all takes about 15 minutes. The top of the implant has a ball much like a mini trailer hitch. This ball fits up into a receiver that has a mini O-ring. This works well to stabilize the denture while waiting for the real implants to heal. The problem is that the minis are impossible to remove after the large implants are complete. They are firmly integrated into the bone.

The dentist decided to just use the minis to retain

the denture. This has become more common. Even I did about 30 of them. I had two fail so they are not foolproof. Both the patients were smokers. It is possible that smoking may have contributed to the failure. Both patients were very upset when they failed because their dentures had been so much easier to wear while the implants were in place. I have recently seen reports that some dentists are placing crowns on these minis. I worry that they may not be strong enough to resist the pressure of a crown in contact with teeth in the opposing arch.

Implants for everything

There is a trend in dentistry that is starting to emerge from all this success. If you go to a surgeon for an extraction, often they are selling you a bone graft so they may place an implant in 6 months rather than waiting for bone to fill the space where the root of the tooth was. Of course there is a charge for the bone graft. These holes will fill on their own. Extraction sites have been healing and filling with bone since the first teeth were extracted. It just takes a little longer, say 9 months.

I had one patient who went to a surgeon to have a tooth extracted. The surgeon insisted on doing the graft even though the patient had no interest in replacing the tooth. Six months later the graft was loose and there was an infection in the area. The graft was being rejected. The patient now needed to have the graft removed and was left with a larger bone defect than if it had just healed normally without the graft. He still does not want *the implant. Surgeons with somewhat elastic ethics insist on grafting all extraction sites. It does add a fee of about $300 per extraction.*

Endodontists, those specialists who do root canals, are getting into the game. Some of the more aggressive among them will look at a tooth that will be a difficult root canal and simply extract it and place an implant. Of course the cost of the implant is about 3 to 4 times the cost of the root canal.

I can understand this if the root canal is impossible but I have a little trouble when it is done just because there is a difficult root canal.

Some restorative dentists also do implants. If they see decay that is difficult and will require extra time to do a crown and maybe an implant, they will do an implant instead. The argument is that the crown may not last, so let's do the more predictable implant. Of course we will never know that the crown will not last if the tooth is removed and an implant is placed. Of course, the implant fee is many times that of a difficult crown and possible root canal.

Implants work, but I fear they are being over prescribed. They are much more invasive and costly than a root canal or a difficult crown.

Who should place implants?

Well, clearly, oral surgeons are trained to do

implants. The problems I have seen are that they sometimes do not align the implants very well. This makes restoring the case with crowns very difficult if not impossible. They also tend to be rougher with the gum tissue and the bone. Periodontists are my favorite implant placers. They tend to be much kinder to the tissue and the bone. Perio surgery is a much more precise surgery than removing teeth.

I think general dentists should place implants. The techniques are not that difficult and the average dentist who is willing to take some continuing education courses and purchase some additional equipment is capable of doing implants.

If you need an implant, I would suggest that you have someone who does 10 a month not someone who does 5 a year. They are technique sensitive. Do not do them just because it is easier to do than a root canal or a crown. While they are very predictable they do occasionally fail.

One of my favorite periodontists started dong implants very early. He was a skilled clinician and a great researcher. He kept careful records of all his implants and followed them for years. When he had a failure, he analyzed and analyzed. One of his failures really bothered him. He kept having the patient back and asking more questions. She finally tired of the endless analysis and said, "I do not know why you are so bothered by this. I lost my first artificial hip also. They had to go to a different material." She had not shared this information with him. Somehow she did not equate the implant for a tooth with an artificial hip. The implants were redone with a different material and it worked.

I had another patient who had an implant done to replace one of his front teeth. The post was screwed down into the implant by the surgeon. However, he did not have his mini-torque wrench to assure that it was tight. I did not know this and placed the crown. It was a beautiful match of color, shape, and size. Two months later, it was loose. I had to cut off the crown so they could torque the post down properly and then do a new crown at no cost to the patient. Two years later, it was loose again only this time the implant had come loose. The implant had to be removed, and a bone graft placed. Nine months later a new implant was placed and 6 months after that I was able to place a new crown. I do not know why this patient still talks to any of us. Remember, not all implants are successful.

VII. The Golden years

HERMAN®

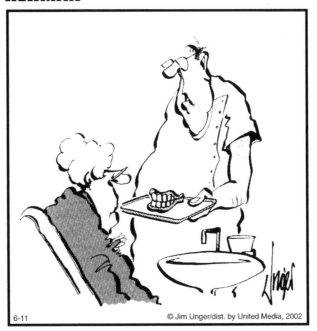

**"These are expensive, but they're guaranteed
up to 140 words per minute."**

21. Dentures

Dentures are much like glass eyes, they look good but do not function as well as the original item.

If you have no choice, you can learn to chew with dentures but it will take time and effort.

Partial dentures

Dentures are a prosthetic device used to replace teeth. There are a number of varieties. There are partial dentures that are often metal with plastic or porcelain teeth bonded to plastic that is gum color to replace missing gum tissue. There will usually be metal clasps that will wrap part way around remaining teeth to hold the partial denture in place. If there are many missing teeth these are much less costly than a bridge that is cemented to existing teeth. A bridge that replaces one tooth costs about 2 times what a partial would cost that could replace 3 or more teeth. Partial dentures take a while to get use to as they are a lot of hardware in your mouth but are much more stable than full dentures.

> *A patient came to me because of her extreme fear of dentistry. She had not seen a dentist in 15 years. I was careful while examining her to not cause any pain. I noticed she had an upper partial denture. I attempted to lift the partial off*

her teeth. I could not get it to move.

I asked her to remove her partial.

She said, I got it 15 years ago and I have never had it out of my mouth.

After bending a couple of the clasps I was able to lift it out. A tooth came with it. Her body had rejected the tooth many years ago. The only thing holding it in place was the partial. I explained to her that it was important to get it out every time she ate and to brush her teeth.

I did complement her on how clean her teeth were. She did a very good job of brushing around the partial.

Partial dentures put some stress on the teeth they clasp. By resting on the underlying gum tissue, they will cause the bone under the gum tissue to be resorbed over years of use. Because of this they need to be relined, refit, every few years. The options to replace missing teeth include fixed bridgework and implants. Both are closer to natural but also many times more costly.

A patient went to a dentist and explained he had saved up for new dentures. He wanted dentures that would work. The dentist examined his mouth and explained that there was little bone to hold the denture. But he had an idea. "Let me drill a hole in the back of your dentures. I will attach about 50 feet of floss to the denture and a piece of bread to the end of the floss. You are to swallow the bread.

The patient asked how that would work. Well tomorrow you will come back, drop your pants. I will find the floss and tie a fish hook to the floss and hook your bottom. That will hold these teeth in place.

The patient said that would hurt. The dentist responded, "any way you look at a lower denture it is a pain in the rear. There is more truth than fiction to this story.

Full dentures

Full dentures replace all the teeth in an arch. As a rule of thumb you can wear an upper denture against lower teeth but should not wear a lower denture against upper teeth. Lower dentures are "U" shaped because there has to be a place for the tongue. Because of this the lower rests on about half the bone that upper dentures rest on. If you have teeth above against a lower denture the force on the lower will cause early loss of jawbone height. Because upper dentures rest on the ridges and palatal bone this is less of a problem.

I had a patient call me one Monday morning. He had been deep sea fishing and had a case of bad breakfast and high swells. He got sick and lost his upper denture over the side. Somewhere there is a fish with a beautiful smile.

He had a very important business meeting that afternoon and needed teeth. His career depended on it.

I went to the office. After all I was a dentist, I could do anything.

I took some dentures I had made on mannequins in dental school. Fortunately, one was about his size. I took a mold of the denture and placed white plastic in the tooth portion of the mold and pink plastic in the gum portion. Before this set, I put the impression in his mouth with the sitting plastic. Once it had hardened, I relined the new temporary denture with a reline material and within an hour he had teeth that would work with a lot of denture paste to hold them in place. His meeting was successful and we made a new set of dentures over the next 3 weeks.

It may be a good idea to have a spare pair in case you lose the others, break teeth, or your dog chews them. This happened twice to one patient and once to several other patients.

Implants

If you have dentures long enough your jaw bones will resorb to the place that it will not be possible to keep your dentures stable. In the past there wasn't much we could do. We now have predictable implants that can be placed in the remaining bone; sometimes bone grafts are necessary to get adequate bone for the implant. Once the implants have healed, attachments are screwed into the implants and the dentures attach to the implants. This comes as close to having teeth as is possible. However, plan on paying $12,000 to $15,000 for four implants and a new denture.

In the last year, we have had mini implants developed. I have done 10 cases. Two cases failed and the implants had to be removed.

The others are all working; several are now 3 years old. The advantage of the mini implants is that they cost about $2400 for all four implants and you can usually use your existing dentures and you are able to use them the day they are placed.

> My first patient came back the day after I had placed his implants. I asked if he had much pain. He said none at all. "I went out last night and had a steak. It was the first steak I had enjoyed in over 5 years. I had pizza for lunch and it did not roll up in my denture. However, I think I will have to sue you."
>
> Somewhat shaken I asked why.
>
> He said, "I am having so much fun chewing I will get fat."

In short, dentures are like glass eyes and wooden legs; they are prosthetic devices and do not work as well as what the good kind Lord gave us. If you have teeth, keep them. If you need dentures you will learn how to use them, but it will take time and they will limit a bit of what you eat and how you chew, and implants can help.

A denture will not cure your dental problems for life. They need to be relined every couple of years and need to be remade about every 10 years. Some people are simply not able to wear them. I have seen people who just could not keep them in their mouths because of their gag reflex. This was prior to implants. I wonder if implants would have helped.

I had a young patient who was in an accident. His jaw bones were fractured and the only way to get them to heal was to remove all his teeth. I built his first set of dentures. Nothing I did worked. I relined them, adjusted them, and encouraged him. Then I did it all again. Nothing worked. I decided I would probably see him once a week for the rest of my life because the teeth fit well and there was nothing else I could do. Implants had not arrived on the scene at that time.

He suddenly stopped coming in. I worried but hoped he had found another dentist who could solve the problem.

Several years later, he was back because he had broken a tooth. I asked how he had been and how they were working. He said there was nothing wrong with his teeth. "I am an engineer and a good one. Because of that they made me a supervisor. I hated it. I had to go to meetings with other engineers several decades older than I. I was very self conscious that I would open my mouth and the teeth would fly across the table. We had a cut back and I am back being an engineer. If they ever make me a supervisor I will quit. I can get another job but I do not have to be a supervisor."

22. How to prepare for retirement

Here is your gold watch;
The retirement party is at 12;
Do not let the door hit you on the way out.
Oh, by the way, your dental insurance ends today.

No Medicare coverage for dentistry

Do you ever wonder why there is Medicare and Medicaid health coverage, but no Medicare coverage for dental insurance? I once visited with one of the elder statesmen in dentistry who practices in Washington DC. He told me the story of how, when he was president of the a major dental organization, he was asked to come to a government meeting representing dentistry about forming Medicare for medical and dental care for the elderly. He proudly stated that he did not believe in government intervention so he did not attend. While he didn't single-handedly defeat the dental insurance bill, attitudes like his are the cause of the problem we have today.

In general, there will be no dental insurance to help with the cost of dental care after you retire. There are a few exceptions. Our state employees can continue paying for their insurance after they retire. Some other unions have similar options. Some plans allow COBRA coverage for a short period of time if you pay the premiums. A few businesses continue insurance for their highest level of management. However, most of us common folk are out of luck.

When I turned 65, I signed up for Medicare. My medical insurance costs dropped from close to $1,000 a month to about $200 a month. But dental coverage is not offered thanks to our civic-minded leader. With the economy being what it is and the cost of medicine escalating at its present rate, I doubt if we will see dental insurance for elderly included any time soon.

A possible partial solution exists

I was interviewed to be a consultant for one of the major dental insurance companies. I suggested they lose about 10% of their members each year to retirement. The last few years are times of high usage as people approach retirement. Why not give anyone who has been on the plan for the previous 5 years the opportunity to purchase their coverage as they go into retirement? They could avoid the heavy push the last few years of coverage and could raise their membership numbers by about 10% a year with little or no advertising. It seemed like a good idea to me but did not impress them, as I did not get the job.

A new idea

A local insurance company is offering dental insurance to anyone for a little over $100 a year. The company pays nothing. They have gone to dentists and offered the dentists to have their name in their book, a list of dentists who will take this insurance. If the dentist accepts this insurance, they agree to do the dentistry for about a 25% discount and the patient has to pay cash at the time of treatment. We have tried this and it is OK. We get paid less but do not have to bill or accept time payments. My guess is we will see more such plans.

Get it done while you have insurance

If you are lucky enough to have dental insurance right now, and are nearing retirement, you have some planning to do. My dental assistant got on my case because I was not pushing those approaching retirement to get all the dentistry done that might be needed in the future, while they still had insurance. I resisted because of my belief that if it is not broken, do not fix it. One patient in particular retired and within a year had 4 teeth break that had large fillings. Could I have predicted this? Well, I couldn't have known they would break so soon, but I certainly did not believe these fillings would survive another 20 years.

Because of cases like this one above, I have since re-thought my approach. We started giving the patients the choice. I explain that I can't tell when exactly, but I can predict that some of their teeth are at reasonable risk of needing a crown. I attempt to prioritize which teeth I think are the worst, so we can do those first. All of this depends on insurance companies agreeing that these teeth need crowns. However, because I am very conservative, my recommendations are usually accepted.

Give the dentist several years to get your mouth ready to retire

If you wish to do some preventive treatment like this, do not go to the dentist and say you are retiring at the end of the month, that you will have coverage through next month, and you want to get all your work done within this time frame. It simply is not usually possible to do it that fast. In addition, most policies have yearly maximums. If you have large old fillings that are breaking down, start getting them replaced or crowned about five years prior to the day you plan on retiring. That gives us a chance to do the work in a reasonable time frame and get as much covered under your insurance as possible.

As you approach retirement, take a good look at fillings that might not last more than a year or two. Do not replace all your fillings as a precaution—that is not necessary. It would be very unusual that all of them are about to fail. Simply replace the ones that look a bit suspect. However, do not come in the week before you get your gold watch and luncheon, and expect me to be able to fix you up by Friday.

Here is the recommended schedule

When to do	What to do
3 – 5 years before retirement	Talk to your dentist about your retirement plan. Mention your time frame. Ask for a thorough checkup of all your teeth that might require attention. Ask your dentist for a treatment plan that will accommodate your schedule and allow you to maximize your insurance. Follow the dentist's recommendation.
1 year before retirement	Verify with your dentist that you are on track. Make any necessary adjustments to your plan.
1 month before retirement	Schedule a checkup appointment to allow the time to take care of any last minute needs and get your teeth cleaned one last time with insurance benefits.

The dental insurance you have is already paid for. Do take full advantage of it while you can.

23. The aging mouth

The new 60 may be the old 40 but the teeth are still 60

I am now a card carrying Medicare recipient. However, I do not feel that old except when I wake up in the morning. Pain is a good sign; it means you are still alive. After a warm shower, the joints work a lot better. However, as we get older we do see some problems that were never an issue 150 years ago. People did not live long enough to see some of these problems. Medical care has improved so much that we are living longer and longer. As a good friend and pharmacologist says, we have really effective drugs. People are living long and longer. The longer they live the more diseases they have and the more drugs they need. Soon they need drugs to counteract drug interactions. Pharmacology is a growth industry. Of course, if you do not to take your drugs you can just die.

Several things happen as we age. Our teeth wear. They tend to crack. The gum tissue and bone tends to recede up the root. If enough support is lost, the teeth can get loose and some may be lost.

There was a time when 50% of the population was in dentures by the age of 50. Now I doubt if it is even 5%. Traditionally, some cultures had all the teeth of young women extracted prior to marriage. In a sense it was a dowry from the bride's parents. In this way the young couple would not be faced with dental costs.

Sensitivity with recession

With much of the population keeping teeth to the time of their death, we see some very difficult problems. As roots become exposed they are sensitive to hot and cold. This can be controlled by using a topical fluoride solution every night prior to going to bed. Get a fluoride gel such as Gel-Kam and after having any food or drink you are going to have before you go to bed, brush your teeth with 4 or five drops of Gel Kam. Swish for 15 seconds and spit the extra out. Do not eat or drink anything. Go to bed and sleep.

You will also prevent decay

The fluoride will precipitate in the microscopic pores of the root. This will desensitize these surfaces. The Fluoride will also harden these surfaces so they are less prone to decay. It is common to see patients in their 80s with decay ringing the necks of most of their teeth. These are very difficult problems for the dentist. Most often it will require a crown to replace all of the tooth above the gumline. This is a problem for several reasons. First, crowns are costly and most people of this age are retired, on a fixed income, and no longer have insurance. It is stressful for the patient and, by the time they are 80 years old, they often have medical issues that make them less able to handle stress. Usually this is not an issue for one or two teeth but often is an issue for the whole mouth.

If everyone who is 60 years old started using a fluoride gel every night prior to bed time, they would spend 30 or 40 dollars a year for the fluoride but they could go the rest of their lives with no new decay. We would not be looking at teeth that were notched the whole way around the root like an aspen tree that met a beaver.

Dentures need to be refit

Those who were unlucky enough to end up with dentures need to have the dentures refit periodically. Typically the denture should be checked by a dentist at least every two years. First to see how the denture fits but also to check to be sure there is no oral cancer. The bone and gum tissue will change but the denture will not. The reline, refitting, needs to be done to keep a good fit. Loose dentures tend to damage the ridges and may cause the changes to happen at a greater rate.

When I see an elderly patient (someone 10 years older then me), the first question I ask before I begin any treatment is, does the dentistry need to be done? What will happen if I do nothing? Is this patient's medical condition stable enough to justify this dentistry and can they handle the stress of the treatment? Am I doing this for them, for their family, or for me the dentist? Is this problem really an issue? Will this problem create future problems for them? Because some dentists operate a for profit atmosphere, it is important for a patient or a family member to determine if a procedure is necessary. Sometimes, a second opinion is a valuable option.

This is age relevant dentistry

I had a patient who was 97 years old. He passed away in his sleep at 98. He was driving until he was 92. He used his rowing machine daily until he was 94. He was a little hard of hearing but in pretty good shape with one exception. He had several molars with decay. Two had actually decayed off one of the tooth's two roots. However, they were solid and he was in no pain. I could have removed the teeth and fitted him with a partial denture that he would have a hard time adapting to. I could take these teeth out and leave him chewing with those teeth that were left. But he was in no pain. He showed no evidence of infection; however, the decayed roots had to have some infection. I would have hated to have him die from a dental infection. I could send him out for implants. It would have been expensive, probably over $8,000 for two implants and crowns. He could have afforded this, but the stress of having this done was significant. I would have hated to have the last years of his life spent in a dental office. I would have hated to have my friend die in my office. He had one further problem. He had a heart pace maker and had been defibrillated once when his heart stopped. He probably was not a good candidate for major dentistry. There really was only one answer to this problem. I sat down with him and his daughter and discussed the problems, options, challenges, and prognosis *of each treatment. They decided that so long as he could eat and had no pain, it would be best to wait and see. Had he lived to 110 and had a dental infection that led to his death, I would know I was wrong. However, it was his heart that gave out.*

VIII. Elastic ethics

HERMAN®

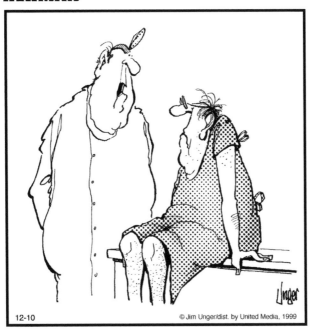

12-10 © Jim Unger/dist. by United Media, 1999

**"Of course your operation is necessary ...
I have to buy a new car."**

24. Paradigm shifts— beware of quackery

**If it looks like a duck,
walks like a duck,
and quacks like a duck,
do not be surprised if it's a quack.**

When I hear the term paradigm shift, my sphincters pucker, and my crap detectors go on alert. Paradigm shift is often just another way to say there is no science, no research, and no validity to what is about to be suggested, but it is going to make me a lot of money as a dentist. In fact, money will be made but it will go the seller not the buyer. When they say paradigm shift, run, do not walk, to the door. Let's look at some of the dental paradigm shifts and think through the problems. Some of these come under the heading of "if it ain't broke, don't fix it".

Air abrasion

Air abrasion came on the scene in late the 1990s. It is essentially a mini sand blaster. A high pressure stream of air shoots tiny abrasive particles out the nozzle. These particles can cut hard tooth structure. Air abrasion is used to clean out the grooves in the occlusal surface (top) of back teeth. It removes a very small amount of tooth, making a groove about 1/2 mm wide (the thickness of 5 sheets of paper).

It is painless

The procedure is presented as not needing local anesthesia. In general this is true, because it is rarely used to cut clear through the enamel layer into the dentine. If a dentist does cut to the dentine, most people will experience pain.

The groove must be filled

Dentists use this procedure to remove the stain from the grooves. When a stain extends down into the tooth it is followed. Once all the stain is gone, you are left with a tooth that has a very thin groove partway through the enamel layer, or perhaps the groove reaches into the dentine. This groove then needs to be filled or food will get into it and cause decay. The filling material most often used is a tooth colored composite.

Most of these grooves will not decay

This sounds reasonable on the surface, but let's looks at what is actually happening. We are cleaning the parts of the teeth that are not normally visible, so the difference is not aesthetic. The claim is that air abrasion prevents decay. But many of the grooves with stain will never progress to decay. I have section teeth that had to be extracted for other reasons from patients in their 80's. The stain goes clear through the enamel to the dentine, but the tooth never decayed. Now if this tooth stayed in the patient's mouth until they were 120, it might have actually decayed.

The vicious cycle of refilling has begun

Once these composites are placed, they will probably have to be replaced every now and again for the rest of the patient's life. We simply do not know how often that will be. And so the vicious cycle begins. Each replacement will end with a bigger hole and the need to be replaced more often.

> *As an insurance consultant I get very suspicious when I see a claim filed on an adult patient with 5 or more single surface composites. This is almost always a case of a dentist with a new air abrasion machine that needs to be paid for. Only extremely rarely do you see that kind of decay in any patient who has had regular dental care.*

I simply am not comfortable opening up grooves because they might have small areas of decay that may or may not be active. If I mess with the grooves, they might get active in a hurry.

In addition to the air abrasion we already looked at, other so called minimally invasive dentistry procedures include the use of very narrow burs to open stained grooves. These may be called preventive odontectomies, preventive fillings, advanced sealants. They are almost always billed out as composite fillings. I have never seen a price break because the fillings are small, easy to do, and require no anesthetic. I have not seen research to indicate there is an advantage to opening up these questionable areas. It is probably better to wait and see. If decay develops, fix it. If it ain't broke, *don't* fix it.

Laser decay finders

A few years ago a device called a Diagnodent came to market. It is a wand that sends a laser light into the enamel and then reads the light reflected back. A computer then analyzes this reflected light and produces a digital readout.

No one really knows exactly what the digital readout means. It is safe to say if the reading is over 50 there probably is decay. No one knows what the numbers mean. There is no unit of measurement attached with the number. If it is under 10, there probably is no decay. Between 10 and 50 is room for a lot of interpretation. It might depend on what your dentist's monthly payments for the device are.

A bit of advice: If you build a box with toggle switches, flashing lights, and a digital readout that is somehow related to the lights and switches, every male dentist in America would have to have one. We are gadget lovers. Women dentists are a little more rational when it comes to gadgets. Now that is a sexist comment.

I had a diagnodent in the office for a month to evaluate. I also had a patient with some small decay is the tops of several of her molars. I could see the decay in x-rays. I checked the grooves with an explorer, a pick, the diagnodent, and x-rays, and compared the results. Sometimes each method was correct. Sometimes each was wrong. Clearly none of the ways we use to check for decay is 100% right or 100% wrong for small areas of decay. Therefore, using several methods in combination is your best bet. If only the diagnodent indicates decay, be cautious.

Lasers

Laser is a magic word in dentistry and medicine. A lot of people want to believe that if it is a laser, it has to be good. There have been studies that show soft tissue cut with a scalpel vs. a laser. You will be surprised that the tissue cut with a blade heals faster. The laser cuts well, but it does so by causing a lot of tissue trauma. The tissue cells actually burst due to the energy of the laser, they are fried a bit like the steak you had for dinner last night.

Other lasers can cut enamel but, again, it looks burned and is not smooth. There are other lasers associated with water that can cut both hard and soft tissues. Those in favor of these suggest local anesthesia is seldom needed. They cure everything from leprosy through canker sores, to traumatic ulcers.

The biggest disadvantage is that these units can be as costly as $100,000. Guess who is going to get to pay for this? In the final analysis, there is almost nothing they do that cannot be as well done conventionally. They are not magic in dentistry.

Controlling the pain of dentistry without shots

I was closely involved with marketing a dental product to do this. In the 1980s a dental product came to market that was to eliminate the need for a local anesthesia, the shot. It was an electronic device. You placed electrodes in the patient's mouth and the patient controlled the current. If they turned the current up, the pain of drilling would go away. It worked, kind of. I did a study on 800 of my patients; about 30% of the time I could drill with little or no pain. But 70% of the time I needed local anesthesia. If I added 30%, a low level of nitrous oxide, my success rate went to about 80%. This was great.

This kind of worked

I started teaching how to use this machine and sold a bunch of them to attendees at my courses. I gave them a great price, about 20% below what the manufacturer would sell them for. In turn, I had to buy 5 machines at a time. They were about $2,000 each. You might say I had a little conflict of interest. In my defense, it was a hot topic and I told the truth. In the end, I found TENS devices that worked the same that I could sell for about $300. They now exist for under $100. I showed my research to all the participants. They knew where it worked and how well it worked. Other speakers only told what the company told them, that it was 90% effective by itself.

It is great to give shots with TENS machines

I did learn a lot about pain control and the neural pathways of pain. I did a lot of teaching. Many doors were opened to me. I even made some money. The one thing that I did show was that these devices worked well to block the pain of giving injections. After treating 800 patients and having about 150 of them fail I noticed that when I had to resort to local anesthesia the patients tended to tell me that was the best shot they had ever had. The light upstairs came on and I decided that I should use the units for blocking the pain of injection. I did some work that showed the patients preferred the electrical to topical anesthesia, the stuff you rub on the gums, 4 to 1. I still use my units for that.

Now for the really goofy stuff.

Piling vitamin in the navel to determine daily dose

I once attended a meeting on alternative techniques in dentistry. One technique that was described was to treat a variety of problems from ingrown toenails to migraine headaches and all areas of the body between these two extremes. The speaker suggested that large doses of vitamin C would cure all our ills. The question was, what was the dose? They demonstrated on a volunteer from the audience. The "patient" was asked to lie down on a table, much the same position they would be in, in the dental chair. They were asked to pull up their shirt to expose their navel. They then clasped the hand of a second volunteer standing alongside of them. The lecturer had the second standing volunteer put their right arm at their side and to hold it as tight to their body as possible.

The lecturer then pulled on this arm trying to lift it. Remember the standing volunteer was holding the hand of the volunteer who was lying prone. Vitamin C tablets were placed in the navel of the volunteer who was lying down and the standing volunteer's strength to resist their arm from being raised was tested as the "dose" of vitamin C was increased. When the muscle testing showed an increase in strength for the standing volunteer it was decided that was the amount of vitamin C, piled in the navel, that the prone patient should take every day.

I had consumed a glass of wine with lunch. It lowered my self control and I had to leave the room laughing. To say there was no science demonstrated may be the understatement of the century. Some of the dentists in the room probably took this technique home to their offices.

Crossing the meridian

There are others who believe in Polarity Therapy. They believe our body is a base of energies that can make us well or sick. They believe in synergy that can create a balance in the body. This can be achieved by deep tissue points rhythmical rocking manipulations, passive unwinding, and gentle holds. This results in mental clarity, renewed vitality, and greater awareness. Some of this group believe the waves of energy can be broken up by crossing the midline of the body with metal. A bridge that crosses the midline must not be metal. A partial denture must have two bands crossing the midline to keep it in balance. Even orthodontic wires must always be in pairs if there is to be balance.

Neuralgia Inducing Cavitational Osteonecrosis (NICO)

There is a theory that much, if not most, facial pain, and even disease far from the mouth, is caused by cavities in the bone, called cavitations. These cavitations cannot be seen in x-ray, CT scans, PET scans, MRIs, or any other imaging techniques. The obvious question of how do you know they exist if you can't see them by using any of the imaging techniques doesn't seem to bother proponents of this theory. The theory further states that the cavitations are infected but cannot be treated by antibiotics. There is a new group of dentists on the scene that do know how to treat these. They call themselves biologic dentists, holistic dentists, or naturopathic dentists among other things. They are also called a number of names that cannot be used in polite company.

This non-problem is costly to treat

I have seen claims come in for as high as $6,400 to drill 4 holes in a patient's jaws to take out samples of bone and rinse the area with antibiotics. In many of these claims, the dentists also took out several teeth with good root canals because these root canals were also poisoning the system. The bits of removed bone are sent to the one and only oral pathologist lab in the whole nation that believes in these. With the exception of this one pathologist, no other pathologist believes NICO lesions can exist in the jaws because of the great blood circulation in these bones.

If you fear you may be suffering from NICO, I would encourage you to read http://www. quackwatch.org/01QuackeryRelatedTopics/ cavitation.html

C Reactive Protein (CRP)

I saw CRP for the first time in 2005. When you have inflammation, your liver creates C Reactive Protein (CRP). You can test for higher levels of CRP. Some studies show an increase in CRP levels after a heart attack. Some folks also suggest that CRP is elevated with coronary artery disease. Some are going even further, suggesting it is causative for coronary artery disease. Some consider elevated CRP to be a positive risk factor for coronary artery disease. Research into this area continues, and hopefully soon we will have a solid understanding of the relationship between the CRP and heart attacks.

Periodontal disease is an inflammatory disease, and therefore it is conceivable that it might contribute to elevated CRP. So far we have said nothing controversial. But now for a giant leap of faith. Some dentists suggest that the periodontal disease causes coronary artery disease. There simply is no evidence that this is true. Those dentists with flexible ethics will sell you nutritional supplements to help control CRP, periodontal disease, heart disease, rheumatoid arthritis, lupus, vasculitis, ingrown toe nails, falling arches, dandruff, and other problems best discussed in private.

Here are a number of web pages that disagree with me.

http://www.perio.org/consumer/happy-heart. htm

http://circ.ahajournals.org/cgi/content/full/ 103/13/1813#F4

http://www.unc.edu/news/archives/nov00/ deliar111300.htm

http://www.eurekalert.org/pub_releases/2003- 01/uocd-uds010903.php

http://www.ada.org/prof/resources/

pubs/adanews/adanewsarticle. asp?articleid=841%20

http://www.perio.org/consumer/mbc. diabetes.htm

http://www.perio.org/consumer/women_risk. htm

http://www.electronicipc.com/JournalEZ/ detail.cfm?code=02250010740815&cfid=&cfto ken

Masters of the obtuse statements

If you follow the research, you will notice that there are a lot of maybes, may, possibly, mights etc. In other words, the large majority of the medical community acknowledges that much is still unknown. One or two of the authors say CRP causes heart attacks, but they do not back this up with research. Note that those with the most to gain are more positive when linking periodontal disease as a cause of heart disease.

As we mentioned, there are two aberrant genes that have been shown to be responsible for an altered inflammatory response. This response is at least partially responsible for refractory periodontal disease, cardiovascular disease, and early deliveries. Each is a marker for the other. If you have one, there is a greater chance that you will have the other, but there is no evidence to go further than that. CRP is the liver's reaction to the inflammatory response. I have not seen good science to show that CRP can cause the problem; I have seen only that its concentration is higher in the blood if inflammation exists anywhere in the body.

How to lose weight with a mouth full of plastic

I had a visitor to my office. She was pushing a weight loss device. She was quite slim. Either it had worked for her or she made a good image as a spokesperson. I had to sign a letter that I would not divulge the design of the device. If I ever prescribed such a device I would first pay almost $3000 and then some monthly sum. For this payment they would do some advertising announcing that I could help with your weight loss program.

The concept and design was based on flawed logic. A patient who was quite svelte claimed her secret was the large bony bump on her palate known as a tori. She simply could not eat fast. I have patients with similar oral manifestations who are overweight.

Because I have been fighting the battle of the bulge all my life, I am always looking for an aid to weight loss. Alas, I have yet to find an effective one. If there was an easy solution I would be there in a flash. I do have news for you all. If you have not fought your whole life to keep off unwanted pounds you will not get into heaven, at least not on the first try.

Breath treatment centers

In the 1990s, dentists started breath treatment centers. They assessed your breath and sold you Oxyfresh. I checked out one local dentist who pushed this. His website stated that he had found this product through a "Paradigm On-Line Catalog (there is the P word again) in the "Oral Health Care" section, ordered a supply, and still, 13 years later, continues to be amazed at the beneficial results his patients experience. As the company grew and introduced other "state of the art" products, he became actively involved as an Oxyfresh Independent Distributor. Does pyramid scheme come to mind? Another ad read "ORAL IRRIGATOR OXYFRESH HYDROMAGNETIC NEW GUARANTEED in the Health Beauty, Oral Care, Systems, Kits category on eBay." Not only oxyfresh but also a hydromagnetic guaranteed product. Just call me suspicious.

Toothpaste with coenzyme Q10 or tablets of coenzyme Q

This is a new one. It is claimed that coenzyme Q is a powerful antioxidant that is good for your gums. You can purchase it from your health food store. I cannot prescribe it because it has not been tested and shown to work. It just is. From the natural food store web site "Coenzyme Q10 is a vitamin-like powerful antioxidant nutrient naturally found in every cell in our body. It is necessary for the production of cellular energy, which is essential for every single process of life."

This probably explains why at 65 my hair is graying and I am stiff and sore when I wake up in the morning. I have never taken coenzyme Q. I think pain is good when I wake up in the morning. It indicates I have another chance at being perfect. I lived through another night and just may make it through another day.

Remember health food products have almost no regulation. No one certifies that the contents are effective. No one checks to see if they are properly processed. St. Johns Wort is harvested by folks who find it in the fields. No one checks to see if what was collected is, in fact, St John's weed.

My wife has made me take Echinacea. Indians used Echinacea to treat snake bite and other poisonous bites and stings and even toothache. None of these were an issue for me. My wife believed it would ether help me avoid the flu or checkout early. (I had lots of life insurance at the time.) I still caught the flu but did have some interesting dreams. The dreams may have had to do with the single malt scotch I used as a sleep aid while suffering with the flu. I do not think the scotch is a cure but it does make the flu a little more tolerable. Echinacea has been shown to have no effect on the flu. I hope no one does a double blind placebo controlled study of the efficacy of single malt scotch.

We seem to see new breakthroughs in dentistry

come our way every year. Most of them go the way of the Edsel, the Mastodon, and T-Rex. I have a closet shelf full of devices that were going to make me more money, make my life better, help my patients, and solve problems that needed solving. The only problem they solved was what to do with my excess cash and how to transfer it quickly to the person who was selling these devices.

We will see new devices and new cures again and again. Some few will work, many won't. I can't cover it all in this book. Be on guard so you don't get intimidated into buying a pricey gimmick or have some costly treatment done with no science that makes your problems worse or worse yet causes a problem you did not have prior to the treatment.

25. Avoiding unnecessary dental work

"Put your hands down, stupid.
This is not a stick up; he is an aesthetic dentist"

You are at your dentist's mercy

One of the areas where a patient is at the dentist's mercy is the exam and then treatment suggestions. We take x-rays, sometimes photos, and possibly models. Then we make a diagnosis based on all of this and present our findings to the patient. The patient is totally dependent on our honesty. No one looks over our shoulder to be sure what we are recommending is truly the best for the patient. And sometimes the recommended treatment is not needed.

Historically, when you sought dental treatment you were offered only those services that were necessary. Times have changed. Many practitioners now offer the necessary work in addition to the ways you can improve your looks. And because people have more disposable income, and because a perfect smile became the newest American Holy Grail, many dentists offer treatments that might not be necessary.

Don't get me wrong. Most dentists are honest and hard-working. But unfortunately, some are not. All you have to do is pick up the Sunday newspaper supplement of any large city to find ads for aesthetic dentistry and smile makeovers. Or go to a supermarket in an upscale neighborhood and pick up a glossy brochure about dentist A, B, or C who is an expert (self-professed) in aesthetic dentistry. Lately, we have seen TV ads several times a night during prime time. These are very, very costly advertising.

You have the right to informed consent

A good dentist will follow his/her suggestion with informed consent. What this means is that you will be told what treatment you need, what treatment is good to have but not absolutely necessary, and what the dentist can do if you like to make changes for aesthetic reasons. The dentist will also tell you the pros and cons of each treatment, the cost, and the longevity of each option. You should also be informed of the risks for all the various treatments. Realistically, if the chance of a problem is very small and the problem is not serious, it probably will not be discussed. We could spend 8 hours mentioning all possible outcomes, the tooth may break, the filling may break. You may be numb for several days to a month if I hit the nerve with the needle. If the potential problem is severe or there is a greater chance it should be discussed, you could die of anesthesia complications; it happens to 1 in 700,000 but it is a very severe outcome if it happens to you or one of your family members. I could break a root canal instrument in the root canal. This happens maybe once a year, but the tooth usually survives. I like to let you know it can happen but the outcome is usually successful. If we do a crown your nerve may die. This is fairly common but does not have a drastic outcome. You should also be told what will happen if you do nothing. If your dentist doesn't do this, ask these questions.

Most outstanding dentist

Pick up *Seattle Magazine*, *New York Magazine*, *Dallas Magazine*, and check out the ads. If they have a yearly dental issue, check out the ads there. Often the ads will claim that the dentist was chosen by peers as being the most outstanding dentist in their area. But in my 42 years of dental practice, I have never received a ballot to determine who the most outstanding dentists were. I don't know of any surveys, or any other mechanisms that would allow dentists to choose the best dentist from a specific area. It is the magazine that proclaims them the best. You will notice that often those allegedly chosen as the best have multi-page ads. Do you think that just might influence the magazine?

Newspaper advice columns

You will find in daily newspapers a section on medical advice, including dental advice. Many readers send in their questions, hoping for good advice from a pre-screened specialist. What the readers often don't realize is that the professionals featured in this section actually pay to be there. This is hidden advertising. Several TV stations even choose a dentist to be their channel's poster dentist. I was once offered this position. It would only cost me $3700 a month. That is over $40,000 a year! I declined.

Marketing can be very costly

I once met a marketing person who told me the marketing budget for one of these aesthetic practices was over $300,000 a year. All of this adds up to a big boost in cost for the dentist, and the cost is passed on to the patients in the way of higher fees. Trust me, aesthetic dental offices have astronomically high fees. If your dentist is spending this much on marketing you can almost be assured they are overtreating, they are suggesting crowns when fillings would work. They are suggesting replacing fillings that could last years. They are telling you how beautiful you will be, how much more self confidence you will have with a smile make over. You will have many photographs taken of your teeth, mouth and smile, maybe even some glamour shots. Your crowns will cost much more than your friend's crowns. I have seen single crowns come into the insurance company at $7,000 when the going rate was $800. No, it was not an error; I called to check. Your dentist will be practicing in a downtown office building, in a plush office and/or in an affluent neighborhood.

The aesthetic courses, institutes, schools

How do dentists get to become "aesthetic experts?" There are various groups and institutes around the country that charge $3000 to $5,000 for a 2 or 3 day weekend course. Some of these institutes actually advertise and recommend that patients look for dentists who have taken their courses. They claim these dentists are in the top 5% of dentists. Actually, about 5% of dentists have taken one of their courses, so it seems that all you need to do to be the best is attend one of these courses. However, no one has ever flunked out. The selection process has more to do about writing a tuition check than ability.

The attending dentists bring their own patients and are somewhat supervised. One dentist gave a patient 22 cartridges of local anesthesia at such a course, when the maximum dose is 10. So the supervision is not that close. This is close to two times the maximum dose of this anesthetic. I would think one of the supervising dentists at the class would have stepped in.

Moreover, some of the instructors have credibility issues. For example, one dentist who speaks at one of these groups has been before the licensing board and was cited for 13 drug violations, from prescribing drugs for non-dental uses to prescribing narcotics for himself. This is one bad example but he has been on staff and has spoken for two different aesthetic makeover programs. No one seems to check credentials.

They learn among other things how to market aesthetic dentistry

A large part of some of these training programs is how to market cosmetic dental services and how to sell these services to unsuspecting patients. Much as my co-authors were nearly scammed. A few years ago, the *Readers Digest* sent a reporter to dental offices all over the country, including some dental schools. The reporter was told several conflicting things by these dentists. Some dentist found the reporter needed just a couple of fillings, another maybe one crown, and yet another a full mouth of crowns. The fees went from under $1,000 to over $30,000. While some discrepancies are to be expected, a range like this is hugely suspicious.

What can you do to protect yourself?
First, insist that all your treatment be sent to your insurance company for predetermination before any dentistry is started. You will need an exam and a set of x-rays. Then wait until you hear what the insurance company will cover. This is a free second opinion.

If you hear from your dentist that they do not do that, that it is between you and your insurance company, you pay the dentist and the insurance will pay you, that they do not get involved with insurances, run, do not walk, to the exit.

If you do not have insurance and you are looking at several thousand dollars worth of dentistry, go to a dentist in a more modest neighborhood. You might have more luck with a dentist who is a little older and who has the kids through college, and the car paid for, someone who does not have a half page ad in the phonebook, someone close to retirement. The opinion from this second dentist will cost a hundred dollars or so but you can save thousands, preserve tooth structure, avoid hours in the dental chair. Plus, you might meet a great dentist.

If your initial exam takes an hour or more and you have models, x-rays, and have photographs taken, be on alert. Be even more careful if they blow up these photos on TV screens, particularly if they are flat screens, to show you "cracks," "failing fillings," "cracks," "bad grooves," "cracks," "thin cusps," "cracks," "leakage around silver fillings," "cracks," "lots of work your previous dentist did not see" particularly if you have not needed much dentistry in the past. Do not run, sprint to the exit.

The ADA weighed in on the side of the dentists

The American Dental Association was incensed that such a thing was done and that it was published. There is always some variation of diagnosis. This is true but from $1,000 to over $30,000? I think not. They should have been concerned that some of their members were taking advantage of their patients.

Insurance companies provide a second opinion

I have seen hundreds of patient records sent to an insurance company for many unneeded crowns. Of the cases I review, 30 to 40% of proposed work is not needed. The patient would be better off not having the work done. I have a network of 50 dentists I can send patients to, to be examined in person. Ninety-five percent of the time, they agree with my opinion.

You might find it shocking that insurance reviews are about the only second opinions anyone ever gets. Of course, if a treatment is rejected, the treating dentist will tell the patient that the insurance company was trying to save money. But that is not necessarily so. The groups I work with, Union Welfare Trusts, are very well funded and pressure me to approve more crowns. But most insurance companies won't cover very expensive smile makeovers.

Remember, the insurance company approval is not automatic. Just because a dentist recommends a treatment, it doesn't necessarily follow that the insurance will pay for it. For this reason, it is absolutely essential that you ask your dentist to get the insurance approval before any work is done. Otherwise, the dentist might start the treatment, the insurance company will reject the coverage, and you will be stuck for a considerable amount of money.

Some dentist with elastic ethics will tell the patient that it will be covered, request the patient pay prior to service, and start the work. They do not know if it will be covered, but once it is started it must be completed. Patients get the sad news that it is not a covered expense months later when they find out the insurance they have does not cover 4 implants and 4 porcelain crowns as happened to one patient. The patient would be out over $16,000 in today's fees.

Craze lines (cracks) are not necessarily evidence of weakness

If your dentist tells you that you have cracks in your teeth and that they are about to break, be suspicious. By the time you are 50, if you shine a bright light through your teeth, you will see craze lines in most if not all of your teeth. These "cracks" are not necessarily an indication of weakness. The enamel can look like a crack without being weak. I describe it as taking a handful of pencils and using epoxy to glue them all together. If you whack this with a hammer, you might break a pencil, but the epoxy holds everything together. Tooth enamel has a similar structure. Craze lines are an optical defect, and not necessarily a functional defect, so they are not a reason to crown a tooth.

The tooth may break but probably will not

Many dentists will take an intra-oral video camera and show you these cracks and tell you the tooth is about to crack. The problem is there is no way to tell if a tooth is about to crack. The tooth might last decades or it might break tomorrow. If it cracks, get a crown then, and you are no worse off than you would have been if you had gone ahead and crowned the tooth. It does not make sense to crown teeth that might crack, because they might not crack. In my 42 years of practice I have seen maybe 8 teeth that cracked so far down the root or between the roots that they couldn't be saved and had to be extracted. The odds are very good that you will not be the 9th tooth to crack in such a way that it will be lost. Other teeth can crack and be lost even though they have crowns, so even a crown is not a guarantee that the tooth will not break.

CTS, Cracked Tooth Syndrome

The trick to watch out for is "cracked tooth syndrome". You can tell yourself if you have this problem. Your teeth will be very sensitive to bite. If this happens to you, go to a dentist and have them take it out of occlusion, which simply means the dentist will grind the tooth down a little bit, or about the thickness of a sheet of paper, until it doesn't touch the opposing tooth. I have a tooth that gets sore about every 5 years. I have it adjusted and it is comfortable for another 5 years. So, the first step is to get the tooth adjusted. After this treatment, paint some fluoride gel on the tooth every night before you go to bed. If after this treatment your tooth settles down, it is not cracked. However, you may have to use the Gel-Kam for 6 weeks to see the effect. If the pain goes away, you do not have cracked tooth syndrome. If the pain gets worse or does not get better after 6 weeks, the tooth is cracked and needs a crown. Hot and cold sensitivity is not a valid indication. The Gel-Kam is a much better and much less costly way to treat sensitivity than a crown.

Once I had one dentist send in for 5 crowns, all for cracked tooth syndrome. I think he had a boat payment due. The only way to crack 5 teeth at the same time is to have the parachute fail to open, or something equally drastic.

The most outlandish submission I ever saw was a request for 5 crowns. The dentist wrote a letter describing the patient who had "buzzing emulating" (his choice of words) from her fillings. The dentist claimed this was a documented phenomenon and the only solution was to remove the silver fillings and replace them with porcelain crowns.

I wrote back. Whatever you do, do not touch those fillings. Have you evaluated the buzzing for frequency shifts or pulsation? There could be an embedded message and if you remove these, mankind will for all time lose this channel of communications with the great beyond. The insurance company would not send this letter back to the dentist, so we suggested a referral to an ear doctor for the patient and a psychiatrist for the dentist.

Silver fillings are safe

Silver filling have been getting a lot of attention. Silver fillings are more properly called silver amalgam fillings. A dental amalgam is a mix of mercury, silver, copper, and zinc. Elemental mercury is toxic in high doses.

There was a boxer who decided he would be stronger if he had mercury, metal, in his system. He injected several C.C.s of mercury IV. The last I heard, several years later, he was still OK. Obviously the brain was not functioning too well prior to the injections.

With mercury locked up in the amalgam, there is no evidence that any one has ever been harmed by silver fillings. It has been studied by the Center for Disease Control and by the National Institute of Health and declared safe. However, some of the salts of mercury can be toxic and some people have made a jump and now refer to the fillings as poison.

As a child when you got a cut or scratch they were painted bright orange with mercurochrome or merthiolate. Both are anti bacterial agents and as such are a bit toxic. Other than the desire to write this book, I survived these administrations of a mercurial compounds with no ill effects. There are also inorganic salts of mercury that are very very toxic. A bay in Japan was poisoned by a chemical company that dumped these into a bay. However, this has nothing to do with silver fillings. Every home has table salt. Table salt is sodium chloride. One is a very explosive metal the other a very poisonous gas. However we all have it on our table. However, no one is trying to ban table salt.

The courts in 2007 refused an appeal to overturn the FDA's refusal to ban amalgam.

I had a member of one of the anti-amalgam groups come up to me and start telling me how irresponsible I was to use silver fillings. I explained to him about table salt and how the mercury was locked up in the amalgam. He said to me, "I do not use table salt, I use sea salt." Clearly he still takes his dumb pills.

The anti groups have even gone so far as to make it impossible to flush the grinding from amalgam fillings down the drain. It did not hurt the patient, how can it be a problem to flush. As a result, getting rid of amalgam fillings requires expensive equipment. Anti amalgam folks say it is so poisonous you cannot flush it down the drain so how can you put it in people mouths? Remember it has never harmed anyone.

The anti-amalgam folks are well organized and well funded

There are well organized, well funded groups opposed to silver fillings. They come to boards and claim the fillings cause everything from leprosy to ingrown toe nails. There is no evidence that any of this is true. If you want to know more go to go to http://www.quackwatch.org/01QuackeryRelatedTopics/mercury.html (see restorative dentistry for a more complete discussion)

Wisdom teeth removal

Third molars, or wisdom teeth, removal is probably the most common unnecessary treatment. Dr. Freedman named these a FUN extraction (Functional UnNecessary extraction). Only about one wisdom tooth in 10 will ever become a problem, yet having wisdom teeth removed is the American way. You turn 16 and get your drivers license, and have your 3rd molars removed often at the cost of over $3,000. It is a 7.5 billion dollar a year business doing unnecessary extractions. In America this is the standard. This is not done anywhere else in the world. In fact, other countries look at this custom as barbaric. For the full discussion of wisdom teeth, See Chapter 17.

Periodontal disease

It has come to light that advanced, refractory, periodontal, gum, disease is a genetic disease. If you got the two bad genes, you have a high probability of having periodontal disease, regardless of how well you take care of your teeth. These genes change the way your body handles inflammation from irritation. This exaggerated inflammatory reaction causes early bone loss. The irritation of bacteria and food left on teeth and calculus deposited on roots irritates the gum tissue. This causes an inflammation, reddening and swelling of the gum tissue. This reaction causes the loss of bone around the teeth. These two genes and this exagerted inflammatory reaction may tend to cause early development of plaque in your arteries. This can lead to heart disease. There is some evidence it will cause pregnant women to have premature deliveries .

Many dentists have taken a quantum leap and decided that getting a person's teeth cleaned will prevent heart problems and premature deliveries. This simply is not true. All three problems are caused by the same two genes but the tooth problem does not cause the heart disease or the premature delivery problems. There are many, many research projects that have tried to show a cause and effect relationship. So far in 2007 none have shown tooth cleaning to prevent the other two problems. If getting your teeth cleaned would prevent your heart attack, no one would put off going to the dentist.

Who's protecting you?

The disciplinary board will occasionally get a complaint about a dentist who decided the patient needed a bunch of crowns. The patient goes to a different dentist who says no crowns are needed. The patient gets upset and files a complaint with the disciplinary board. Will the dentist be sanctioned? Go to Chapter 2.

How do you tell if you are getting good advice or if excessive dentistry is being proposed? If you saw the dentist advertising on TV, be cautious. If you saw them in *Seattle Magazine* or similar magazines, do not take it at face value. If you found brochures in the supermarket, think again. If you have been seeing a dentist for years with little or no dental needs and all of a sudden your new dentist tells you that you need massive treatment, get a second opinion. I believe the biggest indication to get dentistry done was going to a new dentist. Your previous dentist had been monitoring the fillings as they got older. **If it ain't broke, don't fix it.**

Supervised neglect

Some dentists will call this supervised neglect. In fact, it probably is an indication of a caring dentist who only does the work that is necessary. It has also been shown that where the dentist practices is a valid indicator of chance for over treatment. In affluent neighborhoods people get a lot more dental treatment than in poorer neighborhoods. Do you really think that rich people have worse teeth?

What I have seen all too often is: A patient goes to a new dentist. The new dentist looks at the old fillings and says they all need to be replaced with crowns, inlays, onlays, porcelain etc. The work is done and suddenly 10 to 20% of the teeth die and need root canals. "See?" says the dentist, "if the old dentist had done these sooner they would not have died." In fact, if the new dentist had left well enough alone, they might have gone years with no problems. One of my patients went to such a dentist. He replaced all her silver fillings with tooth colored fillings. Everyone one but one of these teeth ended up needing root canals. When she came to me, she had one left without a root canal. I suggested leaving it alone. "Let's see if it will settle down if we give it a few months." It did and she did not need another root canal. Unfortunately, if she had left her silver fillings alone, she would never have needed the root canals.

Get a second opinion

It is always appropriate to ask for a second opinion. It is sensible to ask what happens if you do not get the recommended treatment and how long it will take for this to happen.

If the dentist gets defensive or upset, walk away. It's your mouth and you have the right to understand all the options. Remember, there are few things in dentistry that have to be done immediately. One possible exception is suspicious tissue that could be cancer. Of course if you are swelling, in pain, and running a fever, you are infected and need immediate treatment.

One of the cases I reviewed once made no sense. The dentist wanted to crown some teeth and then extract them. I could not figure any reason for this. I called the dentist and asked him what he was dong.

His response was that he was a Christian dentist.

"That is good," I said. "I am glad you have a faith but what are you doing to this patient?"

"I am a quality Christian dentist. I do not have to answer such questions," he responded indignantly.

I guess that means all my Jewish and Buddhist dental friends must for all time be relegated to mediocrity. He hung up on me. Thankfully, the insurance did not pay for his nonstandard technique.

I would like to close this section with a quote from a dentist I found on the internet.

"Of course dentists overtreat. If dentists did not overtreat, the industry would collapse and what would patients do then?

26. How to avoid shoddy and excessive work

"Trust me. I am a doctor."
Shoddy dentists and overtreaters will only give you one option, the one they prefer.

Ask your friends and expect to be given options

This is a difficult question. The best way is prevention. Research your potential dentist. Ask for a CV or at least a resume. If they have one, it will tell you a lot about them, but not every dentist has one. Ask friends and neighbors about their dentist. Does the work last? Is the office neat and clean? Is the staff friendly? Does the doctor answer their questions? Does the doctor give treatment options along with pros and cons of each option? Shoddy dentists and overtreaters will only give you the option they prefer so they can make the most money. Just call me cynical.

Get a second opinion

It is reasonably easy to look at a crown or a bridge and know if it is well done if you are a dentist. It is almost impossible if you are a patient. If you are concerned about the work you have had done, get a second opinion. If there is a dental school near where you live, it is an excellent option. If you live in a small town, it might make sense for you to go to a different town, so you don't talk to your dentist's golf buddy. However, in many areas that are less populated, the dentists will all know each other as they all go to the same dental meetings and dinners. Ask the new dentist to describe all the work they see you need and explain what they do or do not like about your teeth and the work you have.

The old beat up fillings are the king

Obviously fillings that are over 20 years old will be a bit beat up unless all you eat is pablum. However, a 20-year-old filling that is a little beat up is a good filling. It has lasted 20 years and if left alone it might go another 20 years. They can look very bad if an intra oral camera is used and the image is flashed on a 20 inch flat screen monitor. Those flat screens pay for themselves in short order.

What if your crown comes off

How about crowns that come off? It does happen occasionally. I have one patient who has managed to take a crown off 6 times, she claims 7. The preparation looks good; it has parallel walls that are more than adequate to give good retention. The cement we use is one of the new super strong cements. She does not appear to be a clencher or grinder. I do not have a clue about why the crown seems to come off every 4 to 6 months. She is very good natured and teases me that we have to stop meeting this way. Six or 7 times was probably 5 times too many. I just redid the crown at no cost. I will eat the lab cost. (I am proud to report at the time of publication the crown has been on for more than a year.)

I have many crowns that have stayed in place over 30 years. There are other crowns that simply were done on teeth that were mostly gone. I warned the patient that we could have problems. Some do have to be re-cemented every year or so. I could do gum surgery to get more tooth to grip but having to recement every 2 to 4 years seems a better solution than the surgery. If the dentist warns you about this possibility and then it happens, you cannot claim shoddy work.

We will all occasionally have something fail

An important indicator of the quality of the work is what the dentist does after the problem occurs. A good dentist will work with you to remedy the problem. We all make mistakes occasionally. What you do after you discover you screwed up or that it did not come out the way you planned, is almost as important as the fact that you made an error. When I would get a superior attitude growing up, my mother would remind me that there was only one perfect man and remember what they did to him.

Once a patient called with a complaint. He had moved about 40 miles away, and his new dentist did not think his crown fit.

I asked if he could come in when he was in the area and let me look. He did and I was appalled. It really had a poor fit. I explained that I was embarrassed and would like to do it over at no cost.

He said, "I knew you would do that. That is why I came back."

I redid the crown at no cost and apologized. We remain good friends.

Sometimes it is not the filling or crown that broke

Often a patient will come in with a filling that broke. I first look at the chart to be sure I did the filling. I then look at the filling. If it is broken, I redo it at no cost if it is less than 5 years old. Often the filling is fine, and it is part of the tooth that has broken away. I will get a mirror and show the patient, or I will take a photo so they can see if it is in the back and I can't use the mirror.

Veneers are not forever

When we get into the area of veneers and how well they last, it gets very difficult. If a front tooth breaks, we will often try to repair it with one of our composite materials. Sometimes the amount that broke off just does not leave enough tooth to get a good bond. It may be worth a try to repair the tooth, but I warn patients and write in their charts that I think this might not work. If the repair breaks, we then have to go to a crown, or possibly a more encompassing veneer.

I had one patient I did 3 veneers for. She was a clincher, but I thought veneers would work and it was more conservative to do veneers than to cut the teeth down for crowns. She knocked off two of the veneers about 4 times. I gave up and did two crowns. All the new work was at no cost to her. She felt she had lost confidence in me. I certainly understand why. On the other hand, I got her a strong restoration. She turned me in to my licensing board. They looked at what I had done and what I had done after the veneers broke and decided that what I had done was correct. She called 4 years later after she broke the 3rd veneer. I called her back and offered to do a crown rather than a veneer as we had done on the first two teeth. She never called back.

Dentists should be responsible for failed dentistry

The point of all this is if something goes wrong in a reasonable amount of time, the dentist should redo it at no cost to the patient. A possible exception would be a patient who demands some treatment that the dentist does not feel will work. I had a patient who needed a crown. He wanted an all porcelain crown rather than a metal and porcelain crown because he felt the metal in the metal and porcelain crown would upset the electrical activity of his body. I explained that I did not feel an all porcelain crown would be strong enough as he was a clincher. He said that was what he wanted. So I wrote a note in his chart that I believed a metal and porcelain crown would be stronger but he insisted on all porcelain. Further, if the crown broke, there would be a charge for any redoes. I had him sign the note. When the crown broke 3 years later he decided when he paid for the second crown to take my advice.

Dentists cannot guarantee their work

Do dentists guarantee their work? The American Dental Association claims it is unethical to do so, and in some states it is also illegal. It is also unwise because you never know what the patient might do with their teeth, crowns, and veneers. Clenching is expected; biting ice is not. Biting apples is acceptable, biting fingernails is not. Biting spaghetti is OK, biting thread or plastic bags is not. Patients who will not brush will get decay. On the other hand, while I do not guarantee my work, I redo anything that breaks, provided the patient was not doing something they should not have been doing, or had something unusual happen. I did a porcelain bridge and the patient came back 2 years later with the porcelain gone. A bicyclist had run into her and her face had hit the sidewalk. While I was sorry this happened to her, that really was not my fault.

To summarize, select your dentist wisely on the recommendation of other patients. Take the dentist's advice as to what will work. If you go to a very low cost dentist, remember they may be taking shortcuts. Their lab work might be going out of country. You often will get what you pay for if you go low cost. That is not to say you will get high quality if you go to a spa dentist. If in doubt, pay for a second opinion.

Go back to the dentist or get a second opinion

Let's say you feel what you got done was not correct. What should you do? Go back to the dentist and complain. Give the dentist a chance to make it right. If the dentist refuses, gets insulting, or ignores you. First, ask yourself if you are being fair. Was the crown done 10 years ago or 10 months ago? If you don't get a satisfactory response, go to another dentist for a second opinion. Make it clear you are requesting a second opinion and not an exam that will lead to treatment. The biggest indication to replace fillings is going to a new dentist. Ask what is wrong and take careful notes.

Check to see about peer review before going to the licensing board

Contact the local dental society and see if they have a peer review program. Many problems can be solved at very little loss of time or money with peer review.

File a complaint with your state board/ commission

If there is no peer review or if you are dissatisfied, you can file with the state licensing/disciplinary board. The board will review the case and decide if the dentist was wrong. In a few states this board really is a good old boy's club, but most boards are quite the opposite. They are appointed to protect the citizens and they take this responsibility very seriously. Many boards will include laypersons. These are usually quite helpful.

Take legal action

The last resort is to go with legal action. If you choose this route, hire an attorney. The truth here is that very few problems in dentistry result in a settlement large enough to justify legal actions. The cost of a lawsuit may be many times what you can hope to gain from a settlement.

I have a good friend who is a malpractice attorney. I asked him if he had ever done a dental case. His answer was that by the time he spends 6 months to a year preparing for a case, he probably knows more about the problem than the doctor and he will win the suit. It is not worth his time unless the potential settlement is going to be close to a million dollars for him to take on a case, if he is to get paid for the time and effort he and others will put into a case.

Prevention is the cure

The solution to bad dentistry is much the same as the solution to decay. Prevention is the answer. If you select a dentist wisely, you will not have to worry.

IX. Dental insurance

27. My dentist does not accept my insurance

It says here, to collect on our dental insurance, you are to put the tooth under your pillow and the tooth fairy will leave a dollar bill.

In the good old days, no one had insurance. The bad news was that all dental care cost money, and many people could not afford what they really needed. So, they went without, which was not a good solution. Now, a lot of people have dental insurance, and yet there are still problems. In this chapter, we will examine some of the issues you might encounter with your insurance.

Dentistry is big business

In 1999 dentistry was a 56 billion dollar business. In 2010 it is projected to be a 109 billion dollar business and 167 billion in 2015. Roughly half of this is paid by private health insurance plans. Dentistry is only about 5% of all health care.

Types of insurance

There are 4 chief classifications of dental insurance plans: Fee for service—the more I do the more I get paid; Preferred provider—pay them less than they are worth; they can make it back on volume: Capitation—pay a low fixed fee per patient per month, expect all dentistry to be done for that fee - pay them even less and give them all the risk; Direct reimbursement—they can do anything they can convince the patient to accept and it will be paid without a review up to a yearly maximum.

Fee for service insurance — The more I do the more I get paid

With the advent of dental insurance starting about 50 years ago, people had their employers paying part of the cost. When I was first in practice in 1964, we started seeing plans that would pay up to $1,000 a year for a family, which was the equivalent of about 10 crowns. Life was wonderful for patients and for me as a dentist.

Overtreatment raised is ugly head

The plans paid a percentage of costs for crowns, usually 50%, and 70% of the cost of fillings up to this maximum, no questions asked. The dental insurance companies quickly realized there were some occurrences of overtreatment. Dentists were doing crowns that were not needed and some dentists felt every crown needed a buildup. One company said 90% of buildups were done by 10% of the dentists. The insurance companies started requiring that we send in x-rays as evidence of need.

Fee control

This form of insurance is about 40% of all insurances but the percentage is decreasing every year. Typically the plan will accept fees up to the 90th percentile of all fees and then pay a percentage of that fee. So if 100 dentists file their fees they will accept the fees of all but the top 10. About 80% of dentists sign up for these plans. If your dentist is not a member of one of these, either their fees are high or they simply do not believe in insurance. This usually means their fees are in the top 10th percentile. Remember, fees have more to do with where you are treated than either the quality or necessity of the dentistry.

Insurance helped patients and dentists

Still, having this insurance available was truly a huge step forward. I was able to do treatment that in the past I had not been able to do. People started saving their teeth instead of having them removed because of pain and lack of funds. Initially, the blue collar worker had insurance while the white collar workers were expected to take care of their own. The unions were better negotiators than the professional organizations. With time, all got similar benefits. Then things stagnated. By the mid 70s the maximum was the same but the cost of crowns had more than doubled. But still 5 crowns were not bad and insurance started paying for orthodontics for children of employees.

All of this is in pre-tax dollars

All of this came as pre-tax dollars. If the patient had been paid the money, they would have had to first pay income tax before they could pay their dental bill. As time progressed there was a greater push by business to control cost. We started to see different types of insurance.

The patient will have a co-pay but dentists tend to be happy with these plans because they pay better. It is easier for a patient to find a dentist who will accept this type of insurance. However, because fees are higher and the insurance pays only part of the cost, patients' costs are higher than other plans.

Preferred Provider Organization, PPO plans – pay them less than they are worth. They can make up for it in volume.

About 15 – 20 years ago in the late 1980s, PPO plans arrived on the scene. These are about 40% of all plans; about 50% of dentists sign up for these plans. These plans are increasing at about 5% a year. The plan works as follows: Dentists have to sign up for these plans. In turn, their name is listed in the book given to the patients covered under these plans. The plan can help keep a dentist busy but the profit margin is controlled.

Fee control

The deal was simple. Dentists would accept the plan's patients at a 10 -20% decrease in fees and they would be listed in the plan's book as accepted dentists. If the PPO plan increased the number of patients in the chairs then the deal was tolerable. Or if the employer was a major source of our patients we really did not have a choice. If this happened all at once, and the company was a major employer in your area, a practice had a choice, join or risk losing large numbers of patients, not seeing new patients from this company and possibly losing friends who worked for this company. Not much of a choice.

Some offices say NO!

Some offices said no way, they would not sign up. If they are handsome/beautiful and very charismatic, they could get by with this and not lose too many patients. But the majority of dentists signed up, either out of fear or out of necessity.

Join or your patients lose

The insurance companies had yet a new trick. If you were a participating dentist they would pay 60% of your fee for crowns. So there was a 20% discount and they paid 60% of the discounted fee. An example in today's fees is a crown costs about $1000 or $800 for a PPO plan. Of the $800 the insurance covers, 60% or $480, leaves the patient paying $320. If you went to a non-participating dentist, their fees tended to be higher, say $1200 per crown. The insurance company would base their pay on the average fee, $800, and would only pay 50% of that fee, so the crown that the nonparticipating dentist charged for ($1200) would be paid at $400, 50% of the allowed fee of $800, leaving the patient paying $800 rather than $320. This is because the patient chose to go to a non-participating dentist.

Other considerations

The non-participating dentists screamed discrimination. The plan was a way to help control costs for insurance companies and, to an extent, the cost to patients. What does it mean for the patient if their dentist does not accept their insurance? It may mean their insurance fee schedule is badly out of date and is too low to work with. It can mean that the dentist has very high fees and is so busy they do not have to worry about losing some patients.

High fees do not guarantee quality

In short, you lost big time if you went to a dentist who was not a participating dentist. Remember high fees do not guarantee high value. Fees correlate more closely with where the office is, than the quality of the dentistry done in the office. Offices in the affluent neighborhoods charge more than those in modest income communities. The amount of dentistry you need is often correlated to going to a new dentist and not your actual needs.

The low fee shift to more dentistry

The patient will have a harder time finding dentists to accept this plan. They will not be the spa type practice as the fees are lower and there is less profit to provide these additional amenities. The out of pocket expenses for the patient are lower. However, some dentists will throw in extras to make up for the lower level of coverage. The offices who accept these plans tend to be larger and less personal, or they might be run by young dentists looking for more patients. They will tend to be in the less affluent neighborhoods.

The bargain fee practice or a high fee practice

How can you tell which is the case? In general if your dentist is in the affluent suburbs or downtown in a high-rise building, you can be fairly sure that their fees are high. Look at the office. If it looks like Taj Mahal, someone is paying for this. Ask your dentist why they do not take your insurance. If the answer you get is something like "I am interested in doing only quality dentistry," be suspicious. There is no reason quality dentistry can't be covered by insurance. If they sit you down and show how big a discount they face and show that other insurance companies accept their fees you may have poor insurance. Check around and see what other dentists charge.

Often the best affordable dentistry is in modest neighborhoods

The most affordable, good quality dentistry is often found in the older, modest income neighborhoods of large cities. The folks who live here often do not have a lot of disposable income. They cannot afford excessive costs. Nor do they expect spa type offices. These patients want their dentistry done at a reasonable cost. They do not expect massages, roses, wine, or coffee. They do not expect original art on the walls. They do expect good dentistry at a fair fee. If you want to be over-charged in the high tech neighborhoods, go where there are homes priced at over a million dollars.

We know of an orthodontist who charges $10,000 for every orthodontic case. In addition, you have to go to a different office for your x-rays (more cost). The practice is in a very affluent neighborhood. Three miles from this office in a more modest neighborhood is an orthodontist who taught orthodontics in a dental school for 8 years and continues to teach part time. Her fees are $6,000 per case. A typical ortho case goes on for 3 years and is seen 10 times a year. You save $4,000 to see a better orthodontist but have to drive 180 miles, 6 miles per appointment, times 45 appointments. You can easily determine if this is worth it for you.

Dental Health Maintenance Organization, DHMO, capitation dentistry – pay them even less and give them all the risk

Pay by the head

We next saw capitation dentistry. This means there is a certain number of dollars allocated per patient. This form of insurance is about 10% of all insurance and it is decreasing. Few dentists will sign on for these plans and patients tend to leave once they understand how they work.

How do they work?

We tried some of these plans. We got paid about $45 a month per family. About half the people never came to the dentist. The average family was 2.6 people. We were not required to do crowns if we could do fillings and were not required to do bridges or to replace missing teeth provided the patient had 10 or more teeth. It was "low ball" insurance. Each year I wrote a letter to each family and explained they had other choices and just how much I got paid to see them. The insurance company did not like the letter. I explained my responsibility was to the patient, not the insurance company. After 10 years the insurance company decided they did not want me on this program. Ninety-five percent of the patients switched to the other program within a year to remain our patients. Capitation insurance is much less costly for the employer. The employees like it because they never have to pay anything. However, the patients do not get all the options they get with other plans while on this program.

The dentist is as risk

The offices that take this plan have to be very careful and only provide the services they are required to provide. Some endodontic and surgical procedures must be provided. If these cases are sent to a specialist, the dentist has to pay the specialist. Needless to say, these procedures are rarely sent out.

Plan shortcomings

Some offices tended to make it very difficult to get appointments. Crowns are only done if there are no alternatives. Bridges will rarely be done. The pressure is on the dentist to do those things necessary to assure prevention of dental breakdown. The good news for the patient is there is no cost to them. If they fail to show at an appointment they may be charged. However, they have no choice over what dentistry is provided. They usually will not be able to choose to go to a specialist. This is very limiting insurance and there are very few dentists who will accept it. There is great incentive to cut corners if you are a dentist in one of these plans.

DHMO and PPO closed panels — put the patient at risk

There are a few group practices that are large enough to bid their services to large companies. These typically hire dentists right out of school. This limits what the dentists can do and places high demands on the number of procedures each dentist sees. The young dentist is often placed in the position of having to provide dentistry they are not capable of and excessive demands on how fast they do all procedures.

Problems I have seen

As an insurance reviewer I have seen many complex cases given to dentists that did not have the experience to do such cases. I have seen very low fees for this dentistry, fees so low that I could not come close to providing dentistry at these fees. I see a lot of overtreatment. Rather than one crown, each patient needs multiple crowns. Each tooth needs a build up and crown lengthening. In the end, the fees are just as high per tooth and there are a lot of add-on charges.

Direct reimbursement plans — they can do anything they can convince the patient to accept and get paid without a review

We see a few direct reimbursement plans. You take your bill from the dentist and the company pays for that service up to a certain maximum each year. Some of the dentists quickly figure out that you needed to have that much dentistry done each year.

Reviews control overtreatment

Most insurance plans or union trusts hire dentists as consultants to review submitted cases. I have done this for 15 years. About 50% of crowns and bridges that are submitted are denied for lack of need, or the treatment is outside trust guidelines. I never had any pressure placed on me to keep down costs or to approve less. I often was pressured by the union to allow more dental procedures, as they wanted happy members. They just did not understand that doing unnecessary dentistry was not good for the mouths of their members.

What I have heard from employers

A recent small business, under 100 employees, went from a trust to a direct reimbursement. The trust program was getting more and more expensive. If I cut back the coverage, it would be a negative for my employees, the company would look bad. Their previous insurance paid part of their dentistry, typically 50 to 70% and did not cover some aesthetic procedures. These were seen by employees as being a sign that the company was being cheap. The overall coverage was better because the unused moneys were applied to the overall needs. He went to a direct reimbursement self funded plan. The employee brings in their dental bills and the company pays up to $1500 a year, no questions asked. Very low administrative charges, merely to keep track of what was paid and write the checks. There is no carryover from year to year. Those employees who do not use up their full amount lose it. The money set aside goes back to the company. The employees like the 100% coverage. They would prefer higher limits. The company is saving money.

A possible solution

I made a suggestion to a large aircraft company in our city. I suggested in addition to fee for service insurance, preferred provider insurance, and dental health maintenance insurance that they offer a plan where all treatment is reviewed as to need and appropriateness.

I see a tremendous amount of overtreatment in their present plans when I review the employees' treatments as a secondary insurance carrier. Their carrier did not review most crowns and none of the surgery or periodontal treatment. Conservatively, this review would save the company 50 million dollars a year in unnecessary dentistry, the employees would suffer less and have less unneeded dentistry done and would miss less time from work going to get this unnecessary dentistry done.

I presented this to one of their executives. The company was not interested. Their gross expenditures were so great, 50 million dollars was not worth looking at. They probably spill that much jet fuel each year. I guess I will never understand big business.

A new plan to control costs that works

One more form of insurance is worth mentioning. It was a plan that came with one medical insurance. The company came to us and offered the following: We will add your name to the information our medical insurance patients are given. They are all elderly. You must accept 80% of your usual fee. The patient will pay cash for their dentistry the day it is done. It costs the patient nothing above the cost of their Medicare supplement. It costs the insurance company nothing. The company did not pay the dentist anything. The dentist took a 20% discount but did get paid at the time of service so there was no billing or collecting costs. This insurance made sense. Unfortunately, the company stopped offering the plan after a couple of years.

We are beginning to see this sort of plan again. It is being offered to patients who have no insurance. They pay the company a small fee. The company gives them a manual of the dentists who have agreed to the plan. The patient pays cash but gets dentistry at a discount. That dentist does not have to bill or fill out insurance forms and gets paid the day of service.

Insurance has helped both dentists and patients

Insurance has been the single most important move that has helped the quality of care patients get. In turn, this made my job as a dentist more enjoyable as I could do more and better dentistry. From my experience reviewing insurance submissions, my guess is that 40 to 50% of what is submitted for treatment is either unneeded or the patient would be better off not having it done. It is estimated there is $1,000,000 a day of fraud. The problem is, it is very difficult and costly to prove and prosecute. It is simply easier for the companies to not cover the suspect dentistry.

Who should you ask for answers?

Most patients will not get a choice. Larger companies may offer choices. Before you make a choice ask your dental office and your human resources people. They should be able to give you all the advantages and disadvantages of each plan. If they try to push you into one plan be cautious. If they do not take the capitation plan, do not be too suspicious. This really is pre-paid care by a third party. Insurance is usually reserved for catastrophes where there is big loss but low incidence, auto accidents, home fires, etc. In this case, an employer is paying for dental care that is expected to be needed with pretax dollars.

Dental insurance may be at risk

As the cost of medical insurance rises and it is rising very rapidly, there comes a place where a company cannot afford to provide these perks. If given a choice of losing medical insurance or dental insurance, the dental is the insurance that is lost.

Before you have treatment, review the following:

1. Take a look at your coverage and the fees and services.
2. Talk to the business person in a new dental office and make sure you understand your coverage, reimbursement, and office policy. This really is not considered in dental insurance.

3. You either get insurance or you do not.
4. Negative selection is covered by requiring whole companies to join and limiting the minimum number of employees that will be accepted in the case of small companies.
5. If your company is small, it may be impossible to get insurance. It may also have coverage limitations—what is covered and at what percentage.
6. If your dentist recommends treatment that is outside your plan, take a look at the costs and consider a second opinion.

What is quality dentistry?

The dentist responded to me. "I do quality dentistry. I am a Christian." I have done union welfare trust quality reviews for a number of years but that was a new one. Is this to say that my Jewish and Buddhist dental friends are forever, at best, relegated to mediocrity? When I was in dental school in the 60s, if it was not gold foil, gold inlay or gold onlay, it was not quality. Religious beliefs, however, were not part of our quality criteria.

I felt a great deal of guilt the two years I spent in the Navy. I was only allowed to do alloys, plastics and extractions. I have had a number of dentists include on their insurance submissions a statement telling me they no longer did alloys, in fact, they did not do any metal restorations, they are "quality dentists." Most seem to practice in the affluent suburbs. Here in Seattle they tend to cluster around the Microsoft or other high tech facilities. Their fees are well above average, often two times average. They also find many ancillary procedures to charge for, diagnostic models, photos and night guards for every patient, buildups on all crowns, some even charge extra for impression and temporaries when doing crowns.

These are the dentists revered by dental students and some dental school instructors. I cannot remember the number of students in the ethics class I help teach who make the statement, "I want to associate with a quality dentist with the eventual goal of having a quality practice."

Just what is quality? We in dentistry are just starting to see outcome studies. No one really knows how long different restorations last. Almost no one correlates costs vs. longevity. Does the gold inlay, I was taught to revere, last 5 times longer than the lowly one fifth as costly alloy? Is the direct composite worth 1.5 times the alloy? How long will the composite last? Is the porcelain onlay worth its cost or is this much like most breast augmentation - done for aesthetics with little concern for necessity as opposed to desire.

Are those of us who practice in the inner city substandard? Can "quality" be done in these more modest neighborhoods? Can the dentist who does welfare dentistry hold their head up high when in the presence of "quality dentists?" What is "quality dentistry?"

I have a different definition of quality. I think quality is providing a needed dental service that is well done at a price patients can afford. This places the porcelain onlay used to replace alloys in the same class of a dental aesthetic enhancement, not really needed just desired. Quality is providing well-done dentistry to the low-income patients on welfare where the fees are marginally above what is necessary to pay the overhead of an office.

Quality is giving the patient enough information they can make an informed decision on their options. Quality is a dentist accepting their decision in a nonjudgmental way. If done properly, the patients can be honest about what they can afford and not feel subhuman because they cannot afford the most expensive procedures. Outcome studies tend to indicate that the least costly alternative is often the best for the tooth. Alloy is a very acceptable material. Repairing a restoration may be better for the tooth than starting over and much less traumatic than prepping it for a crown. Alloy (silver) lasts longer and is more cost effective than composites or the newer porcelain onlays and crowns.

In my 36 years of practice, the best quality dentistry I have done, that dentistry I am the most proud of, is extractions. These extractions were done without anesthesia because the patients were afraid of the local anesthesia and would accept pain rather than an injection and the strange sensation of anesthesia. The forceps were wiped off with alcohol soaked gauze between patients. I did these without the aid of x-rays or a medical history. I would lose my license if I did this today. However, at the time I was 3 to 5 miles outside of the defensive perimeter in various small villages in Vietnam. I was the only dentist for about 200 miles. The only dentist these patients would ever see. I know I was the first and probably the last dentist that had ever been in those villages.* All the teeth were badly abscessed and came out very easily. We could only be in the village for about 2 hours for fear of word getting back to the enemy. Post operatively we had a long hot hike home through not so friendly rice paddies with a squad of Marines as protection.** We often had 20 people in line waiting for our service when we had to leave. The old saying of "one tooth in the forceps, a tooth in the air and a tooth in the bucket" was the standard. The only equipment we had was what we had carried with us. You quickly learned to improvise. Yes, this was quality dentistry.

---

* I now know this is not true. American, Australian and probably other volunteer dentists go to Vietnam on a regular basis to provide care. They have even helped start a dental school.

** God I love Marines.

The dentistry I am most proud of is well below the standard of care I strive for in my office today. However, I think the alloys I did today are a better "quality dentistry" than the onlays done by my cohorts in the affluent suburbs doing their aesthetic dentistry. My friend, in his welfare practice, is doing better quality than I. His patients need his service more than my patients do, because there are so few dentists who will do welfare dentistry.*** He should be the dentist held up as an example to the dental students. It should be his statue in the hall of the Dental School. Can you visualize the citation, "A welfare dentist who did his best." He is the dentist we should have been taught to emulate. He is providing the most needed service to the greatest number of patients. He is a "Quality Dentist."

This book is meant as a self help guide to aid you to take control of your mouth, understand your dental needs and treatment options.

Clearly I have not examined your mouth. I have not looked at your x-rays. I cannot even guess what your dental needs might be or what the most appropriate treatment will be.

*** Medicaid, welfare, pays about 40% of usual and customary fees. Overhead, all the costs to run a dental office, is usually above 60% of a dental fee. The dentist dose not get paid, they have to pay to see Medicaid patients

I can only suggest with confidence that you will never be wrong to get a second opinion.

This book is not meant to be a do-it-yourself dental diagnosis manual. It is intended to make you a more prudent Dental Consumer.

How to use the appendix.

Medical history form
1. If your dentist does not use as complete a form, copy this page and fill it out.
2. Circle all the problem areas in red so they stand out.
3. It is very important to be very honest about your medical problems
4. The allergy question is very important. We need to know what medications and foods you are allergic to.
5. Many people are becoming allergic to latex, rubber. This is very important to your dentist as they probably use latex gloves. They can use not latex gloves and avoid other rubber materials if they know you have this allergy.
6. It would not hurt to give your dentist a new copy of this history form once a year, whenever your medical status changes or you start a new medication.

Dental history form
1. Record what type of filling, crown or bridge was done, what date it was placed and in which tooth.
2. In the future if a filling or crown fails you will have a better idea of how long your dental work is lasting.
3. You can ask for a copy of your chart. However, I have reviewed hundreds of charts from dental offices and find many are nearly unreadable.

Drug history
1. It is important that we know what prescription, over the counter, homeopathic, naturopathic, legal and illegal (street drugs) you may be using. The may interact with the drugs we may prescribe.
2. This list will also give us a good idea of what your medical problems are.
3. I would copy this form every time there is a change and give it to your dentist.

MEDICAL HISTORY

NAME_____ Physician's name_____ phone number_____

Circle any of the following that apply.

1. Are you having pain or discomfort at this time?	YES	NO
2. Do you feel very nervous about having dentistry treatment?	YES	NO
3. Have you ever had a bad experience in the dental office?	YES	NO
4. Have you been a patient in a hospital during the past two years?	YES	NO
5. Have you been under the care of a medical doctor during the past two years?	YES	NO
6. Have you taken any medicine or drugs during the past two years?	YES	NO
7. Are you allergic to (II.e.., itching, rash, swelling of hands, feet or eyes) or made sick		
by penicillin, aspirin, codeine, or any drugs or medications?	YES	NO
8. Have you ever had any excessive bleeding requiring special treatments?	YES	NO
9. Have you ever taken diet medication? Which medication did you use_____	YES	NO

10. Do your have Osteoporosis or have you taken the following Fosamax Didronel, Boniva, Aredia, Actonel Skelid or Zometa
    (these are drugs used to treat osteoporosis. They can cause major problems for extractions)   YES   NO

Please circle y for yes for any of the following which you have had or have at the present. Circle n for no if you have never
had this condition or disease. Please circle one or the other for each condition or disease   y   n   HIV AIDS

y n Heart failure	y n Emphysema	y n Hepatitis A (infectious)	y n Fainting or Dizzy Spells
y n Heart attack (MI)	y n Cough	y n Hepatitis B (serum)	y n Nervousness
y n Angina Pectoris	y n Tuberculosis (TB)	y n Hepatitis C	y n Psychiatric Treatment
y n High Blood Pressure	y n Asthma	y n Liver Disease	y n Stroke
y n Heart Murmur	y n Hay Fever	y n Yellow Jaundice	y n Ulcers
y n Rheumatic Fever	y n Sinus Trouble	y n Liver Transplant	y n Glaucoma
y n Scarlet Fever	y n Allergies or Hives	y n Drug or Alcohol Abuse	y n Bruise Easily
y n Artificial Heart Valve	y n Diabetes	y n Hemophia	y n Pain in Jaw Joints TMJ)
y n Mitral Valve Prolapse	y n Thyroid Disease	y n Venereal Disease (Syphilis, Gonorrhea)	
y n Heart Pacemaker	y n X-ray Treatment	y n Genital Herpes	y n Arthritis
y n Heart Surgery	y n Kidney Trouble	y n Cold Sores	y n Artificial Joint
y n Anemia	y n Sickle Cell Disease	y n Cortisone Medicine	y n Rheumatism
y n Congenital Heart Lesions	y n Chemotherapy (Cancer, Leukemia)		y n Blood Transfusion

Do you smoke?   YES   NO   Do you use recreational drugs?   YES   NO

11. When you walk up stairs or take a walk, do you ever have to stop because of pain in your		
chest, or shortness of breath, or because you are very tired?	YES	NO
12. Do your ankles swell during the day?	YES	NO
13. You use more than 2 pillows to sleep?	YES	NO
14. Have you lost or gained more than 10 pounds in the past year?	YES	NO
15. Do you ever wake up from sleep short of breath?	YES	NO
16. Are you on a special diet?	YES	NO
17. Has your medical doctor ever said you have a cancer or tumor?	YES	NO
18. Do you have any disease, condition or problem not listed?	YES	NO
19. Women: Are you pregnant now? YES NO Are you practicing birth control?	YES	NO
Do you anticipate becoming pregnant?	YES	NO

CURRENT MEDICATIONS_____

*To the best of my knowledge, all of the preceding answers are true and correct. If I ever have any change in my health, or
if my medicines change, I will inform the dentist at the next appointment without fail. In case you need extensive dentistry
requiring a series of payments, we reserve the right to request a credit report to guide us in extending credit.*

*Because of HIPAA , Federal regulations protecting your privacy, we wish to inform you we will release no information about
you without your consent. We are allowed to release this information to your insurance company or as necessary to get paid
for our services. You can have access to your records by simply asking. We will give you a copy, if you desire. There is a copy
fee. If you feel we have released information you have the right to file a complaint. The above statement is required by Federal
HIPAA regulations.*

Date_____ Signature of Patient, Parent or Guardian_____ All patients BP____/_____

Yearly up dates - If any changes, please tell staff what the changes are.

Date_____ Any changes YES NO   Signature_____ BP____/____ ASA I II III IV

Date_____ Any changes YES NO   Signature_____ BP____/____ ASA I II III IV

Date_____ Any changes YES NO   Signature_____ BP____/____ ASA I II III IV

(the section in bold is to help the dental office be in compliance with HIPAA regulations. You have a right to have a copy of
your chart and records. The dentist is allowed to charge for copying the record. They can release information to your insurance company to get paid for the work they have done. They cannot release this information to anyone else. You have the
right to complain if they should do this.)

Drug inventory: What do you take, perscription or over the counter

Drug name	Dosage	How often do you take it	What is it for

History of dental treatments

Date mm/dd/yr	Tooth number or letter	surfaces or procedure	material	What was done

208, 231, 229, 232, 233, 255, 214, 224, 230, 130,
132, 250, 255, 256, 119, 123, +

Made in the USA